Cancer - My Rainbow in the Dark

To GRETEl

my Fellow WARRIOR!

Jim Morrison

By Jim Morrison

Stage 4 cancer survivor

Cancer - My Rainbow in the Dark
Jim Morrison

Editor: David Kilmer
Production Design: Jeff Rowley

Copyright © 2016 by Jim Morrison, Post Falls, ID

ISBN 13: 978-1542713818
ISBN 10: 1542713811

Dedication

I dedicate this book to Jack Wooten, my fellow strong and courageous warrior, an extended family member who fought a warrior's fight right up to the finish.

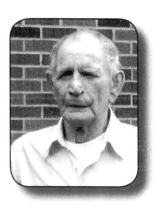

Contents

Foreword

I always ask, "Who wakes up in the morning and says they want to be a cancer advocate, let alone a lung cancer advocate?" Nobody!

My wife, Keasha, was one of the strongest advocates I've ever met. She was a very fit 38-year-old who had never smoked. We were married on Nov. 27, 2011, and one all-too-brief month later, she was gone.

Instead of wedding gifts, she asked people to support that fight. It was my job to figure out how. With Team Draft and the Chris Draft Family Foundation, we are now leading a national campaign to change the face of lung cancer by putting survivors first.

I feel fortunate that I met Jim Morrison at a LUNGevity Foundation's National HOPE Summit after we connected through fellow cancer warriors.

I remember watching as my brave and beautiful wife went from a survivor to a survivor's advocate when she decided she wanted to fight. With Jim, I was impressed that he had taken his fight to a new level by reaching out. He is an inspiration to use our talents to help other survivors.

My wife was a professional dancer, and that's how she connected with people. Through Jim's written words, he is connecting with cancer survivors and their families all over America and the world.

Surviving cancer, for both the person and those around them, takes a never-give-up spirit. You've got to fight for life, and there will be obstacles from financial to transportation to family challenges. If you're not ready for this big ole' fight, it's gonna eat you up.

I love the fact that Jim uses the term cancer warriors. We always make sure to use the word survivor, not just patient. It changes the language, and in doing so, it changes that mindset. Jim knows firsthand. He's been through that battle.

As a retired football player, I know about the warrior's life. To win in football, in life, and in cancer, you must combine physical determination with a smart game plan. You need to be efficient with that plan, be aggressive with that plan, and stick to that plan no matter what.

In cancer, as in football, the injury report is essential to dictating the game plan. Often you would love to call certain plays, but you just can't do it. You must learn how to work with the talent you have available and the injury issues at hand. Yes, be aggressive and determined. You must have that to win. But always make sure you have a game plan, too.

That's where a guy like Jim has been instrumental in so many people's lives. He's not just cheering us on to be warriors, but showing us how to live that warrior's life, how to set goals and beat them in order to survive.

The day of our wedding, my wife found the strength to stand up. She rose from her chair, and stood up to walk that aisle and to dance in my arms.

Now we're asking other survivors to stand with us.

Through his writing and his ministry to others, Jim Morrison is standing up, and I am profoundly grateful for his work.

May this book inspire you and those around you to win the fight of your life, whatever and whenever it might be. I know you can.

-Chris

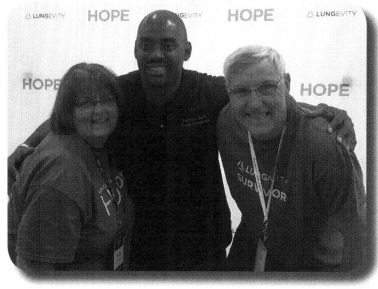

The Colors of Cancer

Most people are aware that a pink ribbon shows support or awareness for breast cancer, but did you know that other types of cancer also have their own associated colors? Here are the most common.

All cancers = Lavender
Bladder cancer = Yellow
Brain cancer = Gray
Breast cancer = Pink
Cervical cancer = Teal or teal with a white border
Childhood cancer = Gold
Colon cancer = Blue or brown
Esophageal cancer = Light blue
Head and neck cancer = Burgundy
Kidney cancer = Orange
Leukemia = Orange
Liver cancer = Green
Lung cancer = White or clear
Lymphoma = Light green
Melanoma = Black
Multiple myeloma = Burgundy
Ovarian cancer = Teal
Pancreatic cancer = Purple
Prostate cancer = Light Blue
Sarcoma/bone cancer = Yellow
Stomach cancer = Periwinkle
Testicular cancer = Purple
Thyroid cancer = Blue/pink/teal (tricolored)
Uterine cancer = Peach
Honors caregivers = Plum

Introduction

Has it really been 12 years since my sudden diagnosis with stage 4 lung cancer?

That many birthdays and Christmases since my family doctor broke down in tears as she brought me the worst news of my life?

Well, my friend, I have a lot to tell you. In that eventful decade, this walking dead man has experienced many things that make me incredibly thankful to be alive. I have danced with my daughter at her wedding and held the new life of grandchildren in my arms. In my stubborn determination to see just one more sunrise, I have celebrated the start of another day more than

WHAT CANCER CANNOT DO:
CANCER IS SO LIMITED...
IT CANNOT CRIPPLE LOVE,
IT CANNOT SHATTER HOPE,
IT CANNOT DISSOLVE FAITH,
IT CANNOT DESTROY PEACE,
IT CANNOT KILL FRIENDSHIP,
IT CANNOT SUPPRESS MEMORIES,
IT CANNOT SILENCE COURAGE,
IT CANNOT INVADE THE SOUL,
IT CANNOT STEAL ETERNAL LIFE,
IT CANNOT CONQUER THE SPIRIT.

4,000 times... and counting. I have watched the sun rise on family vacations, hunting and fishing trips, our favorite place on the lake, or simply through my kitchen window in a moment of quiet gratitude. The gift of that many sunrises is amazing, considering that on January 4, 2004, I was given just six short months to live.

I want to thank all the people who supported my first book, *To See Another Sunrise: How to Overcome Anything, One Day at a Time.* I'm grateful for the many who have read it and recommended it to fellow cancer warriors and anyone else who is struggling in life. I'm humbled when someone tells me, "When my friend was diagnosed, the first thing I thought of was to take them your book." Or when I visit a fellow cancer warrior for the first time and my book is resting on the coffee table full of page tabs. I've received emails from all around the United States, Canada and even Poland. Crazy!

Since then, I've been asked to write again. My thought was if I lived long enough and collected enough real-life stories to complete another book, I would. Well, it didn't take long. These are stories of cancer, both good and bad. I assure you they are all true because I have lived them or have been involved with the warriors who did.

At the age of 50, I began a journey that was not on my list. That

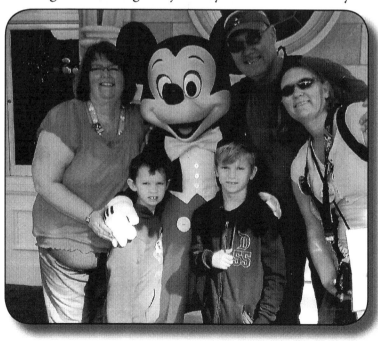

journey left me feeling helpless, powerless and confused, living with severe pain and searching for hope. These things became the "new normal" every day. And yet that journey absolutely transformed me and showed me a life I would have missed without cancer.

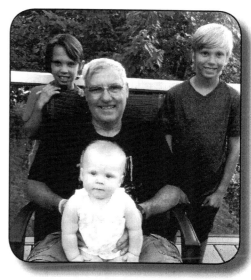

As I write this new book, I feel a calming peace inside as I watch the snow fall outside my office window. Reflecting back, I realize again just how small I am and how huge God is. How faith and hope can see me through the valley of the shadow of death. Every sunrise brings not only a new day, but another sunset to chase.

It's been 12 years since that dark diagnosis, and I have lived the past nine years in total remission with no evidence of disease, thank God. I have twice yearly checkups. The cancer-fighting drug Tarceva®, and all that goes with that wonderful pill, has been part of my life for years. I was the one in 14 that will be diagnosed with non-smokers lung cancer each year. If you have lungs, you can get cancer.

I have found that every cancer and every cancer warrior is different, just like every chemotherapy is different and the side effects will also be different for each person. I have met warriors who died nine days after they were diagnosed, and an 80-year-old five-time cancer survivor who still goes for a walk with me every month.

Cancer is cancer. It happens to the best of us, and all the questions we ask do not change it. I am amazed every time my phone rings or another email connects me with another name. It's crazy how much cancer exists just in my little part of God's world.

I do my best to share my cancer experience with anyone who really wants it. Yet it's surprising how many warriors will not talk about the foe that may kill them. Because that's exactly what cancer wants to do: kill you. This disease is not a broken leg, folks! You can

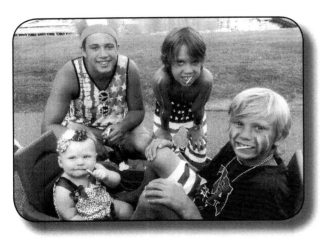

take that lightly and probably still walk again; but not so with cancer.

At best, we have one shot to be tougher than this disease. The question is, are we tough enough?

I've been asked more than once to think about cancer in some other light than as a killer. "That term seems harsh," people will say. The first thing I ask in reply is, "How are you doing with your cancer?" And nearly always, they reply, "Oh, I don't have cancer, my (spouse, parent or sibling) does."

I ask you to go in with your eyes open and don't mistake cancer for anything but the killer it can be. Take a military approach. As one of my best buddies who served in Vietnam told me when I first got cancer, "Jim, it was my choice to serve my country and go to war. Your battle came to you not by choice. In war there will be casualties, but you must fight on to protect and help your fellow soldiers, and remember, in war it is, 'kill or be killed.'"

Harsh? Very! Welcome to the war on cancer.

That first book brought me all the way through my son's wedding in July of 2011, and I predicted their first child would be my first granddaughter. At the time that was my newest goal. Calling things that were not as though they were was my priority as a cancer survivor, just as faith is being sure of what we hope for and certain of what we do not see.

Come with me through the maternity room, living rooms, hospice rooms, ICU and infusion rooms, cancer groups and funeral services of my fellow cancer warriors. It's in these desperate places that real courage appears.

It's said you can gauge a person's courage by how much it takes to discourage them. I will share stories of men and women who, without choice, have been chosen for the fight of their life. Is it bad luck, hereditary, environment, bad habits or lifestyle? In my experienced opinion, we can get cancer in our lifetime no matter what anyone says or does. I believe God can and will allow cancer to break us down so he can renew and retool us. That was certainly the case with me. Yes, I consider myself a blessed cancer warrior. *(Daniel 4:37, NIV)*.

As survivors, our lives are not determined by what happens to us but by how we react to what happens. It's not what life brings to us, but the attitude we bring to life. A positive attitude causes a chain reaction of positive thoughts, events and outcomes. It is a catalyst that creates extraordinary results – a rainbow in the dark.

My life is my message and my message is my life. You may agree with me or not. If you're looking for a politically correct book on cancer, this isn't it. Instead, come with me to the true front lines, as I do my best to tell you the wonderful things God and cancer have instilled in this regular, ordinary retired heating guy.

I am humbled to be able to share with you my thoughts and my heart about cancer. My very existence here today means hope, and you need hope. May we infuse each other with the wonderful power that the one and only God of hope can bring, and together find the good things that cancer can deliver in our desperate place.

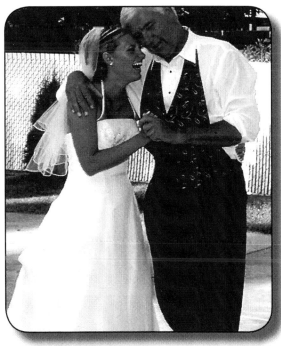

-Jim Morrison,
December 2015

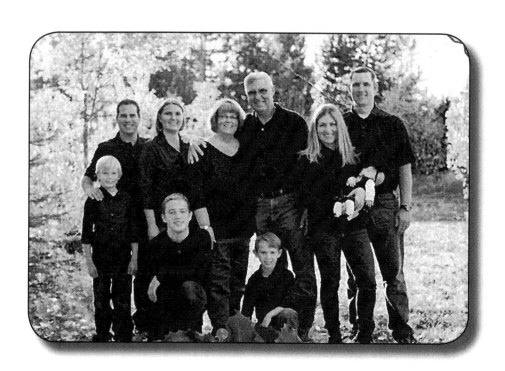

CHAPTER 1

Impossible Goals Achieve Impossible Rewards

What is wrong with me? Why did it take stage 4 lung cancer to make me truly appreciate every sunrise and pursue every sunset? How about you?

It's human nature to take everything for granted. We chase the newest, fastest, trendiest must-have things, whatever they happen to be. We obtain those things just to start complaining again and begin the chase all over. It's never enough to make us happy. We wonder, *what's missing for me to have some joy in my life?* Thank God cancer ended that chase for me.

Cancer gave me back life's true meaning, for which I will always be grateful. I am blessed to have the God of hope in whom my soul finds rest. My hope comes from Him alone. Now all I want is family, health and enough money for what we need, along with that joy deep inside that a new sunrise brings. Today, I am a warrior and a dreamer, one who refuses to give in or give up.

HOPE GOT ME HERE

Tomorrow is a powerful word in the cancer world. It makes us focus on each small thing we need to do to see that next sunrise. As the saying goes, "It's hard to plan your future if you can't get past today."

If you've read my first book, you know how I set goals that helped me focus forward. Without those goals, I found that cancer always made me think about the days before my diagnosis, when health was not constantly on my mind and I had no pain and no worries about the next CT or PET scan. Instead of focusing on the past, I learned to focus on the future. My favorite new goals were based around family: a wedding, a birth, a graduation... one by one, I ticked off each new achievement against all odds.

Family is so very important to the cancer warrior. I rank it number two on my list of important "F words" that helped me win my fight (see them all in Chapter 5). My wife, Sandi, and I are blessed that our daughter, Kym, and our son, Jeff, both married into families who can actually stand each other when we're all together. With me included you know it's a mildly dysfunctional circus, but I will say that this bunch puts the "fun" in dysfunctional.

Cancer requires an X-ray of your family to see what it's really made of. Ours proved what I knew to be true: I have a sound family. All members vowed to be there in my hour of need and to experience our rainbow in the dark together. As the saying goes, "You can gauge the courage of a family by how much it takes to discourage them."

One of many emotional milestones was living long enough to

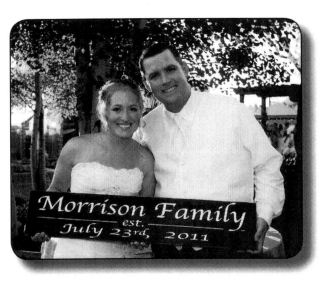

see my son marry his wonderful bride, Stephanie. I remember taking the center floor with Stephanie for our dance, crying and hugging her tight, overwhelmed by gratitude. It was July 23, 2011, six and half years after my diagnosis, with another impossible goal reached.

As Sandi and I watched the newlyweds walk the aisle, I wondered about my future goals. Could I be there to meet my first granddaughter? Perhaps some more grandsons to carry on the Morrison name? Time and fate would tell, but I told myself that, God willing, I would be in that delivery room. As my favorite passage in Daniel 1:8 says, I had "made up my mind."

WITNESSING ANOTHER GOAL

December is a cold and snowy month in North Idaho and any ray of sunlight is welcome. On the weekend before Christmas 2013, what started as a normal dreary winter day turned joyful very quickly. Jeff and Stephanie invited everyone out for a pizza dinner, and handed both sets of parents a Scrabble board.

"What does it say?" I asked Sandi, struggling to read the darn thing

"Oh Jim, brace yourself," she said.

The letters spelled out, "BABY MORRISON DUE IN AUGUST."

After I burst into tears of joy and exchanged high fives and a toast, I immediately set my next goal to be there for the delivery date of August 2014. Would it be a granddaughter as I had predicted at the wedding?

Even as cancer tried to take life away, God brought new life. Earlier in my cancer battle, when my daughter and her husband had given us similar announcements, I was terrified by the thought that I would not live long enough to see my grandchildren born. I learned to turn

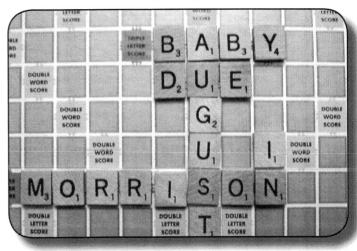

terror into hope and set that goal as another reason to live. I remember reading, "Be joyful in hope, patient in affliction, and faithful in prayer." Against all odds, predictions and statistics, I was incredibly fortunate to witness both my grandsons' births. The victory I felt cannot be bought. At the time of this writing, those boys are ages ten and eight. Thank God I have been given wonderful extended time with them. Another birth provides my latest goal; the chance for another notch in my warrior belt.

Fellow warriors and caregivers, I want you to know that you need a goal; something ahead of you to focus on and strive for. It doesn't have to be huge. Some of my early goals make me laugh at myself now 12 years later: Walking to the bathroom on my own accord; putting on some clothes; eating something; just sleeping; trying not to vomit on the bathroom floor again; not yelling at my caregiver (Sandi); not thinking negative. Some of these small goals can seem impossible, but each goal accomplished will set your mind to achieve bigger and better things.

Spring is always welcomed in snow country. By March 2014, the anticipation of a new season was upon us. Once again, Jeff and Stephanie invited us to a family gathering, this time at a nice restaurant on the river. As we basked in the sunshine on the outdoor deck, we wondered what the heck was going on. Stephanie deepened the mystery by handing out envelopes with instructions not to open them until we all counted down together.

My hands shook as I held that manila envelope with Sandi by my side, my incredible caregiver who had been there with me for all of my health struggles – and some serious ones of her own as well.

"Three, two, one, open!"

The picture inside that envelope brought more joy than we could imagine. I looked at it through tears of joy and with a grateful heart, a sinner saved by grace.

The photo showed Stephanie and Jeff, who is an avid duck hunter, standing in the Idaho wilds. With them were three mallard duck decoys – two big ones and one tiny bathtub-sized one… painted pink. We were having a granddaughter.

Of all the wonderful goals that my God of hope has allowed me

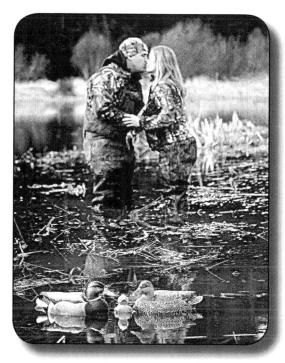

to achieve, the most treasured are the ones who call me Papa. I couldn't wait to welcome this new life.

In middle of the night on August 17, 2014, Sandi and I answered the phone's first ring and sprang into action, driving like maniacs to the maternity ward at Kootenai Health. We raced to the elevator and pounded the button for the second floor. Our son, Jeff, cool but nervous, greeted us with a hug. As we eagerly awaited our first granddaughter's arrival into the world, my thoughts drifted back to the pain, confusion and fear I had experienced on this very floor just ten years before...

DON'T FORGET THE PAIN

I excused myself from the family group, located a cup of hot coffee and wandered back down the hospital hall toward the ICU unit that had saved my life. Back then, I'd spent a lot of time and (very weak) energy trying my best to navigate around this floor. Oh how sick, and how close to death, I'd been. With the toll the deep vein thrombosis had taken on my legs, every step was painful, but still I walked. On our slow struggles through the hallways, I remember Sandi and I peering through the baby window to view new life, both of us praying those precious little ones would be spared from cancer.

Those odds are not good: 1 in 2 for men, 1 in 3 for women. Approximately 43% of men and women in America will be diagnosed with cancer in their lifetime. Please, fund research!

Now, as I walked those halls ten years later, I felt the grip of fear again: What if? Under that old death sentence, even hope and faith had been difficult to find, and I wondered if light would ever shine my way again. One of many lessons I learned in that darkness was not to depend on myself, but instead to trust in the God that raises the dead.

How wonderful were the doctors, nurses and this entire facility. They made a very stressful time bearable. My family lived and slept on this floor for 14 straight days. We shared a lot of tears and gummy bears (my snack of choice during the treatments) and discussed life and how we all take it for granted. Wow, what an experience that had been.

Standing outside the ward like a little lost kid, alone with these deep thoughts, I heard my name: "Jim, we can go in now."

My daughter-in-law was in heavy labor and show time was about to begin. My deal with Stephanie was this: *I want to witness my new and only granddaughter being born. I will certainly respect your privacy, but I paid a heck of a price for this event and I will be in that room.* I chose the corner chair behind the head of the bed. With Jeff now clothed in blue scrubs and ready to assist the doctor, the process was under way.

SET GOALS AND ACHIEVE GOALS

In that delivery room, with my mind racing, I begin to reminisce again. I thought of all the goals I had reached since my diagnosis in 2004. Kym, our daughter, was to be married in seven months. The problem was that I was given six months to live. My first goal, then, was making up my mind to be at my daughter's wedding, and we would dance.

And with our father-daughter dance, I proved statistics and percentages are just that. I proved that faith, hope and attitude can help you to face anything, even against very poor odds. Dancing with the new bride that beautiful evening in July, our feet adorned with black flip flops, her head lying against my shoulder, we found joy beyond description filling our hearts. Doing and seeing the impossible gave me, and everyone around me, hope.

My second goal was surviving to witness the birth of my first grandson. While I was on this critical care floor, soon after one of my surgeries in 2005, Kym brought my new grandson, Byron, (Mr. B) and his older brother, Austin, for a visit with papa. Slim indeed were the odds given to ever meet any of my grandchildren. Nevertheless, holding his warm and precious body close against mine gave me courage to fight on. With a very tough recovery ahead, Mr. B was my fuel to keep going, get better, defeat cancer and prepare my mind for the next goal, whatever that might be. With these impossible goals now notched in my warrior belt, I was becoming more confident about my future. Dear warrior, I want you to know that our best way to predict the future is to invent it, letting faith and hope help us make it a reality.

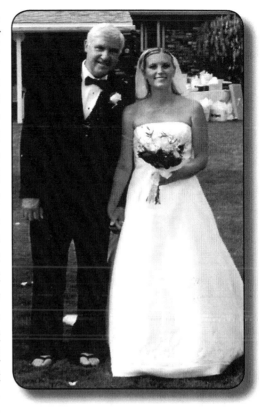

GOING FOR ANOTHER GOAL

I pulled another chair into my corner of the birthing room to prop up my aching legs. Even with compression stockings my legs hurt constantly. *Stephanie is a strong young woman, I thought, giving birth the old-fashioned way. That's courage!*

I smiled to think my baby Jenna was on the way, with everyone waiting for her to join the family, and I was here, too. The doctor was now in the room with us, and I could sense the pace picking up. *Could this really be happening? Was I still alive to witness the birth of my granddaughter?*

As I tried to wait patiently, I reflected back on goal three: to be at my son's graduation.

That morning came with a sunrise never brighter, as I stood with Jeff on his graduation day from the University of Idaho. It was another impossible task completed for both of us. That poor kid had to endure not only a very tough college program, but manage to keep it all in focus while his dad fought the battle with cancer. We both received honors that day, mine coming in a hug and kiss from a very grateful son, who knew all too well the odds I might never have been there that day.

My goals had continued to expand. When Kym and her husband, Jimmy, shared an ultrasound picture of our third grandson on Christmas morning 2007, I could not wait for summer to arrive. How many miracles is one man allowed? This cancer warrior was fortunate enough to witness another one, the day I held little "Carter Sauce" in my arms. What a gift to receive for believing in the impossible. How tiny, but how huge this new life was to a papa so acutely aware of the fragility of my own life.

I believe that life starts with cancer; cancer can make life new again if you allow it. A good mental attitude may not cure you, but a bad one will always make you sick.

OUR FAMILY GROWS

Wow, what a valiant job Steph did giving birth to a new life. Through my tear-filled eyes I could still make out our new grandbaby's tiny body as the nurses prepared her to meet her mother. Her first little cry melted my heart. *Oh Lord, what a tremendous blessing you have by your grace bestowed upon me and my family.* I trembled to know I was witnessing yet another miracle. Here on August 17, 2014 at 3:46 a.m., I was face to face with our newborn granddaughter, Jenna Avery Morrison. Afraid to hold the baby because I couldn't look at her without crying, I excused myself from the room and headed to the east wing of the floor. I retraced my steps around the floor where God had intervened in my life. I wanted to see another sunrise from the hospital, this time not wondering if was my last, but instead with hope and joy in my heart.

I stood in a very familiar spot, the wall supporting me now as it had all those times before. Just down that hall was proof that faith and hope is real.

Jenna, Papa is alive, and I love you. How blessed we are.

Ten years earlier, barely leaving the hospital on my own power, I had no idea that all this amazing life would come my way. I certainly didn't think I'd be around to see it. I walked out that morning ten feet tall as a proud grandfather, knowing the odds were astronomical. Once again, I did not know what my future

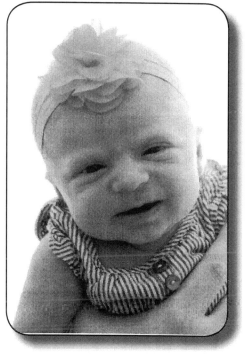

held, but for sure, I knew who holds it. *(Daniel 5:23, NIV)*

My fellow warriors, I pray you experience what only the rainbow in the dark can offer those who find its treasure. I share my story to inspire and encourage you to hold out for just one more goal and one more sunrise. I realize there will be nights that will feel impossible. I know, because I had many of those, too.

Warriors, we must have hope as an anchor for the soul, firm and secure. Your endurance is inspired by hope. We must have faith, reliance, loyalty, and complete trust in God. Now, faith is being sure of what we hope for and certain of what we do not see. After being told my situation was impossible, faith and hope were all I had left.

Come with me warrior, caregivers and all who struggle. Let's walk through the valley of the shadow of death together. Please allow me to share with you the very valuable lessons that God's rainbow called cancer have taught me, have taught us all.

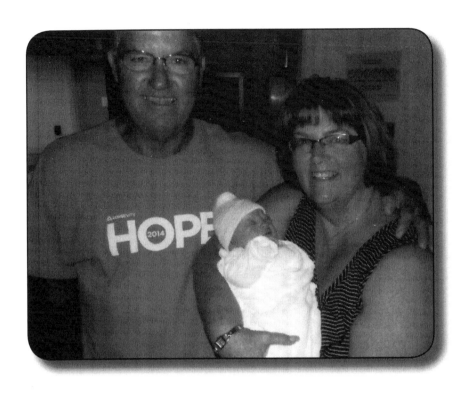

CHAPTER 2
The Lull Before the Storm

My journey with cancer began in the dead of winter, 2004. Our Idaho home was snowed under, and I was attempting to shovel the driveway. For some reason, I really struggled to catch my breath, becoming more exhausted with every stab at the snow. Something was very wrong. Just yesterday, I'd felt absolutely fine and the week before, I'd worked my butt off fixing heaters so my customers could be warm and comfortable in their homes.

I was more tired than I'd ever been. The next morning, I was puzzled by the fact that I couldn't get out of bed. Sandi took me to the ER for a series of tests and lab work, and I was relieved to get back and rest at home. Little did I know we were in the lull before the storm.

After a troubling call from our family doctor, Sandi rushed me back to the hospital. This time, I wasn't going home. As the dark clouds of anxiety and fear rolled into our minds, we became more aware just how unprepared we really were for what was about to overtake us. How do you prepare for something you don't know is coming? Welcome to the world of cancer!

SIGNS OF THE STORM

It turned out my gallbladder was failing, so I underwent surgery. As I lay in the ICU the doctors continued to run tests including X-rays and CT scans. My legs were burning and I couldn't walk. I was nauseous and breathing was difficult. I could feel myself becoming weaker and weaker.

Our family doctor brought more bad news. With Sandi at my bedside, Dr. Susan gave us these chilling words: "The CT scan shows a golf-ball-sized tumor at the top of your left lung. The X-rays show massive amounts of fluid in both lungs and around your heart. We need to extract this fluid right now to relieve the pressure. We have maybe two hours to handle this or we could lose you. Your body is shutting down. Hang in there, Jim."

Now the brunt of our own personal storm was approaching very quickly. After a tearful hug and kiss, Sandi went running from my room, hysterical with fear, to notify waiting family.

I was wheeled out of there at breakneck speed, down to the ICU emergency room where they sat me up to remove the fluid from my lungs. I remember resting back in my own hospital bed, with my two-hour death sentence commuted. I was overwhelmed with joy that I'd made it.

The new day brought a new procedure. The doctors ran a probe down through an artery in my leg and up near my heart. There, they installed an inferior vena cava filter. The idea was to prevent the blood clots now discovered in both legs from traveling to where they could do any more damage.

On January 12, 2004, the shadows of fear, doubt and death made it mighty hard to see another sunrise out my ICU window. I'd been looking through this pane for nine days now. Who knew how many more days I had left? In the midnight hours I felt the storm building and had the desperate feeling that all hell was about to break loose.

THE STORM ARRIVES

My oncologist, Dr. Tezcan, entered my room. My entire family was now gathered around my bed, all sick to their stomachs from waiting so long for any report.

"The results are bad, very bad," the doctor said. "The findings show stage 4 lung cancer which has metastasized to the pericardial sac around your heart. This is rare, and usually does not respond to treatment as well."

"How long do I have to live?" I asked the doctor. "I want it straight, no nonsense."

After he drew a deep breath, he handed me my death sentence.

"Based on my experience and past reported cases of the disease with no response to treatment, six months," he said. "And if you respond to treatment and have no side effects? A year and a half."

How can you ever be prepared for news like that?

THE STORM'S DAMAGE

It turned out I had several serious health challenges. The stage 4 (metastatic) non-small-cell lung cancer had spread to the pericardium around my heart. It was so close that radiation therapy or surgical removal were both out of the question. I needed chemotherapy. I also had disseminated intravascular coagulation, or DIC, a clotting of small blood vessels throughout the body, and often a precursor to massive organ failure. I continued to have cardiac tamponade, a compression of the heart that occurs when blood or fluid builds up in the space between the myocardium (heart muscle) and the pericardium (outer covering sac of the heart). I would undergo surgery for this, as well as a separate surgery for the fluid in my lungs.

All told, Jim Morrison was just about a dead man. But not yet!

Today, I am a 12-year survivor, and I have been NED (no evidence of disease) for nine years. To reach this point I endured 30 months of infusion chemotherapy, two ports installed, two blood transfusions, three relapses, complete hair loss three times, bone shots for blood count, three surgeries, including removing a significant portion of my left lung with the tumor. I've lost count of CT, X-rays, MRIs and PET scans, not to mention lab tests, blood thinners both oral and sub-q injections, and taking my Tarceva® pill faithfully for nine years.

Enough of that medical stuff. All cancer warriors know what's involved, right?

What I really want you to know is the fresh new start that cancer offered me. Since cancer, I can tell you the sunrises are more eagerly anticipated, and the sunsets more spectacular than ever before.

Cancer gave me an entirely new appreciation of how wonderful and precious all of creation and life really is.

Yes, it comes at a very steep price. Are you okay with being a survivor? Of going through the agony to reap the rewards? Cancer leads us into the darkness of desperation, but at the very bottom of its evil pit, I unearthed a treasure and found appreciation. Thank you, cancer!

FROM MY HEART TO YOURS

An extremely intense storm named cancer blew havoc into our calm lives. It arrived under the radar and without detection from the Morrison family's previously serene and stable control tower. Suddenly, there were not enough sandbags available to hold back the tears now flooding our hospital room and our home.

Wow! What a change a day can bring. One day I was a hard-working business owner; the next, a cancer patient forced into early retirement. I had been planning to have a retirement party; instead, now I might be planning my funeral. Just like that, overnight!

The storm analogy seems to best express how cancer came upon me and my family. With now 12 years of experience under my belt weathering cancer storms, my own and others, I have found that most of them blow in unexpectedly. Like the destruction we have been witnessing with our new weather patterns, intense storms like never before are destroying entire towns with billions of dollars in damage.

Here in North Idaho, we experienced hurricane force winds in November 2015. This fierce storm left many homes, businesses and schools in total darkness. Trees that had been around for years toppled. I had six huge trees either snapped in half, or completely uprooted just in my yard alone. Tall and sturdy they stood, beautiful to the eye, but without a good root system to hold them steady in the storm, down they went.

I felt that way after cancer very quickly devastated my family and uprooted my business. Cancer renders us helpless no matter how prepared we think we are. It can quickly destroy and leave, but the collateral damage remains – deeper and more difficult than any physical damage. Cancer shows us what our structure, our root system, is really made of.

I want to share those unseen struggles of cancer, the storms you hear and feel, but may not see. Cancer invites both evil and divine; darkness and light, to a fight in your mind. I guarantee the storms are strong enough to kill.

Never in my life have I been exposed to darkness like cancer brings. I found myself fearful of every little sound, thought and pain, afraid of my own shadow. To survive, I had to go beyond my comfort zone, unprepared and unarmed, into that dark.

I have been through the ultimate storm, my friend, and I can tell you that this fight for our life requires more than human strength and material things. Come with me as we figure out how to fight the good fight together.

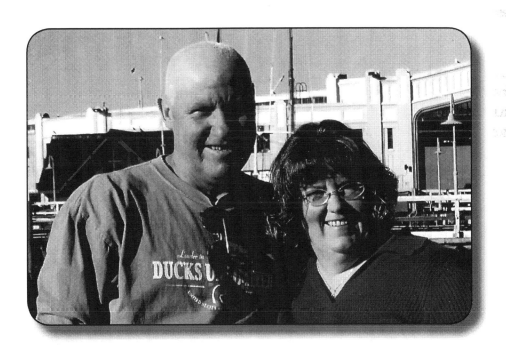

Warrior Words – Jerry

There is a part of me that hates cancer with a fury. It robs us of those we care deeply about. Both in my personal life (wife, father, friends) and in my job as a pharmacist in a cancer center, I've observed its relentless attacks. And yet, I've seen God work amazing good in the face of even this dreaded enemy. I've witnessed His Spirit shine even brighter in the lives of some of those whose bodies were fading away because of cancer.

I think of my co-worker and friend, Dennis, who had drifted in his walk with the Lord and recounted to us how he had prayed that God would do whatever it took to draw him back. He honestly saw his cancer as an answer to that prayer and though cancer in time claimed his life, he died with a beaming face as he seemed to see Jesus in heaven even before he left this earth.

And especially I think of my sweet wife, MaryJane, and how her countenance remained so radiant, so full of Jesus and His life and love, becoming even more striking as her body was wasting away from cancer and side effects of treatments. Witnessing her faith in the face of all she'd gone through helps to strengthen mine and that of many others who observed her.

One expression of her faith is summarized in a thank you note she wrote four years into her battle to a friend who, with sweet intentions, had shared a book with her about that author's experience of healing. Here is that note:

"Thank you so much for your thoughtful gift. I read it while sitting next to a crackling fire with my Bible handy to check the context of the scriptures used. It was a lovely way to spend a morning.

I believe with all my heart that the Great Physician is the same yesterday, today, and forever and that He will heal me. My faith is challenged to trust Him with the timing – whether it's here on earth, or in heaven where there will be no more pain or death. I have peace in knowing that all the days ordained for me were written in His book before one of them came to be. *(Psalms 139:16)* I won't leave this earth one millisecond before God says it's time. It seems presumptuous to tell the Almighty Creator of the universe how He should do things. I choose instead to submit to His authority, purpose, and plan for my life, recognizing that all is grace. Even cancer is His gift to bring me to greater dependency on His strength to sustain me. To Him alone be all the glory! Thank you for kindness and especially for your faithful prayer support."

These were not just idealistic words to her; this was her true heart, cultivated from years of praying to God and reading and memorizing His Word, and she lived it out. I don't want to give the impression that she was just complacently resigned to dying from cancer because the opposite is true; she had an enormous will to live, made all the more intense when she knew there were two more new grandbabies on the way. There were definitely some very hard times and struggles for her, including severe pain and ascites in the last months, but she finished her time in this life so well, focused on totally trusting the Lord.

As her husband, the hardest part for me, by far, was after she went home to heaven and I was left behind. I shared her faith that God is in control and knows and wants what is best for those who love and follow Him, but the emotional, mental and physical grief was much greater than anything I had experienced in my life. The loss of the person in this life who had become so much a part of my own identity and filled so many different roles for me, including being my very best friend that I most trusted and relied on in hard times, was overwhelming.

In my head, I still knew God was in control and had my best interests in mind, but it sure didn't feel like this could be best. But God wants me to remember that what is best for me is not based on how I feel but instead is based on drawing me to depend more on Him, to walk closely to Him, and to be changed to be more like Jesus.

He's trying to teach me to cry out directly to Him (instead of swirling around in self-pity in my own mind) and to look to Him for my sense of belonging and to ask Him to fill the void left in my heart. I'm very thankful that our loving God does answer those prayers.

-Jerry

CHAPTER 3

The Desperate Place

With the sunrise still hours away, I'm staring out my east-facing ICU window at stars trying to pierce the dark. Wide awake, I sense doom and defeat closing in. I'm not sure I can handle this new day coming. Today, I'm convinced, I will be handed my death sentence.

Evil is an artist and cancer is its masterpiece. Evil cancer has me now chained to its dark prison wall within my desperate place located right above my eyes.

Here, while awaiting my sentence of death, the relentless shifting of shadows wears me down, spiritually, mentally and physically. I begin to succumb to doubt and discouragement. I feel abandoned and helpless, ignored, despised and rejected. I am taunted by a vicious and evil enemy and even ridiculed for my faith. I am drained and on the verge of death.

Cancer loves to isolate me into its own bleak corner. Here its evil infiltrates and screws with my mind until I convince myself there's no hope and no way to defeat this foe. To make cancer's day, I find myself here singing the blues of desperation.

Taken captive and all alone, I am in this desperate place where cancer lurks and waits to see what I'm made of. It waits and watches while I stumble, crawling, vulnerable for attack.

Cancer is an animal of prey, looking for opportunity. I must pray so I will not be preyed upon.

I cry out from my pit to God and family. *Why me Lord, why*

cancer? I am only 50 years old. My family needs me. Please release these chains of death. I want to live!

I hear the sounds of life continue all around me. I see so many people but they can't hear me screaming. *Can anyone help me?* My plea echoes off the wet, cold walls for only me to hear, and for evil to rejoice.

How do I respond now that everything in life seems to be defeated? Can I find any hope for good?

In this desperate place, I notice the only book I have in my room. It has somehow been turned over and butterflied open. With nearly all hope gone, I reach for what I hope might give me something, anything, to cope with my deadly situation.

My Bible is open to chapter three of the book of Daniel. I read along, not only to pass the time, but maybe to distract my mind long enough to give it some much-needed rest. Slowly taking in every word, I am caught up in this true story of three young fellows who are defying the king.

These guys are nuts, I think. Don't they realize by disobeying the king's orders he will sentence them to death in a blazing furnace? By now the king is outraged these three young punks will not worship him and obey his order. The king, all high and mighty, questions the young men, "Is it true you guys do not worship my image of gold I have set up?"

The king gives them one more chance to bow down and worship something they hate. He goes on, "If you young men do not worship me, I will have you all thrown immediately into a blazing furnace, then what god will be able to rescue you idiots from my hand?"

(Pardon my paraphrase of the New International Version, but I needed some humor that very discouraging January morning). Alone in that hospital room, taking a sip of water to extinguish my parched, cracked lips, I continue reading.

The three men replied to the king, "O Nebuchadnezzar, we do not need to defend ourselves before you in this matter. If we are thrown into the blazing furnace, the God we serve is able to save us from it, and He will rescue us from your hand, O king. But even if He does not, we want you to know, O king, that we will not serve your gods or worship the image of gold you have set up."

Could I ever be that strong? Regardless of the dire circumstances in which they found themselves, these young men remained firm, unwilling to compromise their convictions, even with a certain sentence of death.

A RAINBOW APPEARS

And with that sudden realization, there in the dark of that dreary morning, the dim lights were transformed into my rainbow in the dark. I looked deeply into this rainbow and I experienced hope in the midst of death. Oh, how that renewed mindset warmed my insides. I felt an unseen force come over me, redirecting my inner gaze from my desperate place to one filled with light.

I still can't fully put into words what this early morning read did for my morale.

When my oncologist walked into the room that morning, I was sitting up straighter in bed, now prepared to handle my sentence of death because I knew in whom I trusted.

And even if he does not rescue me from cancer, I will not bow down and worship its evil.

I was standing firm, without doubt, ready to allow faith and hope to create my future. Thanks to those three devoted young men who had given me hope, I had been delivered to a place of strength and understanding

FINDING THE POT OF GOLD

I now understand why my pot of gold was found only in my desperate fight for life. The rainbow only shines through the dark, and that rainbow is a promise of a new start, a second chance to get it right this time. I believe your own treasure will also be found in the direst of your circumstances.

Listen! The darkness qualifies you to be a survivor. A seed only grows after it is buried in the darkness of soil. Only in the darkness of a blazing furnace will you really find what and who you believe. Only there, in your very worst circumstances, will you truly be able to see the brightest light.

At the end of that story, King Nebuchadnezzar leaps to his feet in amazement and asks his advisers, "Weren't there THREE men that we tied up and threw into the fire?" They replied, "Certainly, O king." He said: Look! I see FOUR men walking around in the fire, unbound and unharmed, and the fourth looks like a son of the gods."

As you well know, I believe in Jesus Christ. Why? Because he was perfect and still faced problems. In fact, he experienced that desperate place.

Yes, the Lord himself agonized in the garden. His desperate place led him to the cross. Do you realize that the darkest moment in the history of man was the afternoon Christ was crucified on that cross? Darkness covered the entire land for about three hours in the middle of the day. All nature seemed to mourn over the tragedy of the death of God's Son.

Only from his most desperate, darkest place did Jesus become the light of the world. "The people living in darkness have seen a great light; on those living in the land of the shadow of death a light has dawned." *(Isaiah 9:2)*

Because of that day and His experience in a desperate place, you have a choice to make. To whom do you turn when things go bad? Do you choose light or darkness? Heaven or hell?

How do we ever overcome such an evil enemy as cancer? Blind it with light!

HOPE SHINES BRIGHT

Early one morning, while I brewed a big enough dose of coffee to fuel my writing session, a newspaper headline caught my eye: *Body of Missing Country Singer Recovered at Lake.*

I read the story and recoiled in shock.

He was a fellow hunter who had been duck hunting alone and had evidently fallen overboard into icy waters. Although he managed to swim to shore, he had finally succumbed to exposure.

Yet the story had a powerful ending. His publicist said; "Thankful to know he fought his way from the water to a hill and was lying in the shape of a cross looking up to his Heavenly Father…"

Fellow warriors, I have "made up my mind" *(Daniel 1:8)* to choose the hill I will die on. Of this I am sure: the same God who created me wants to join with me in my worst times. He is willing to run, walk or crawl with me all the way through the furnace, the cancer and the valley of the shadow of death.

I want you to understand that this survivor shared the same dark feelings and struggles you have. "To whom much is given, much will be required." *(Luke 12:48)* I wrote this book to shed light and offer hope in the darkness of your desperate place. As a cancer survivor, I say this in utmost humility, "I am hope for someone."

When cancer calls, it bids us come and die. I was so very afraid, not knowing what was in store. Death casts a frightening shadow over us because we are entirely helpless in its presence. You must know that the shadow of death cannot kill you, like the shadow of a dog cannot bite. However, under this shadow of death, truth is much distorted in its darkness. I pray this for all my fellow warriors, "Let the light of your face shine upon us, O Lord. You, O Lord, keep our lamp burning, God turns our darkness into light." *(Psalm 18:28)*

THOSE BIG, BAD D'S

When cancer had me by the throat, I found that every terrible thought, word, feeling or image started with a "D."

Of course Jim, you dummy, "D" for death.

No! Not so fast!

Here are cancer's devious "D" words that troubled me so. If we can understand them, then we can, by God's grace, overcome them.

DOUBT: *Is there a God? If God really loves us, how could a loving God allow cancer? I will never be a survivor.*

DISCOURAGEMENT: *My problems are overwhelming. I will never see my goals come true.*

DIVERSION: *I don't want the right things anymore – I want the wrong things.*

DEFEAT: *I have cancer and my life is over. Why me? Why should I even try?*

DELAY: *I'm going to put off anything and everything – including the big decision that could impact not just my earthly life – but my eternal life.*

DISABLED: *Cancer's mind games tell me I am beaten. There's nothing I can do.*

Fellow warriors of cancer – or of anything else in this tough life of ours, don't let the "D" words beat you. Stay true to what you believe, even in that most desperate of hours. That choice alone can change the darkness into the brightest of new days.

"The Lord himself goes before you and will be with you; He will never leave you nor forsake you; do not be afraid, do not be discouraged." *(Deuteronomy 31:8)* My hope is that you will be delivered to a place of appreciation, strength and understanding. May the Light of the World help you to overcome, instead of being overcome.

NOTES FROM THE FRONT LINES
Warrior Words – Raydeane

"You have thyroid cancer." Those words are as clear to me today as they were in 2004 when I was diagnosed. At 37, I was already a breast cancer survivor, mother of two elementary age children and neck deep (no pun intended...well maybe) in the chaos and beauty that is life.

It wasn't as shocking the second time around, but equally as sobering. Adjustments would have to be made and my schedule was now subject to change. My body would go through some challenges that I wouldn't be able to control. I distinctly remember an idea interrupting all the scenarios racing through my heart and mind: *"This doesn't have to be a bad thing, Raydeane."* I call those moments "conversations from heaven." Because honestly, who on earth would think that way?

It shifted my perspective of this new reality. Instead of worrying about how the cancer was going to negatively affect my body and my relationships with the people closest to me, I began to meditate on the new pathways and possibilities that were about to become part of my existence.

And, really, this is the paradigm we all are faced with, in the various game-changing situations of our tenure on earth. None of us escape pain. Each one of us will come face-to-face with a trial or challenge that seems too great for us to bear. The question isn't if, it's when. Our thinking shouldn't be *"Why?"* (why me, why this, why now), but *"What?"* (what is the lesson to be learned, the new epiphany I would have never had without this detour?)

I'm a big proponent of positioning yourself when trouble hits. You have to figure out where you're going to stand at the beginning of a trial. You pretty much have to assume, whatever is going on, is for your benefit. Also, that you are deeply loved by your Father in Heaven. That He is not only aware of your circumstance, but watching over it carefully and mindfully. The first thought that wants to invade your space during tough times is: *What did I do wrong? Does God not love me? Has He forsaken me?* That kind of thinking is not a strong place to battle from. Instead, fight from the position of being set apart and hand-picked for your specific dilemma. Strength will come, fortitude will go before you, and perseverance will be your banner. Just think! You are going to learn lessons from that "secret place." You are about to be a wealth of information, encouragement and hope for many, many people.

You've got this!

I would be faced with yet another diagnosis in 2008: melanoma. As I listened to my dermatologist telling me what my new life with this disease would look like, the voice over the phone began to fade away. I heard the familiar still-small voice, with comforting words and tender mercies whispering in my ear: *"Everything's going to be okay, Raydeane."* I could literally feel my feet firmly planting, my face setting strong like a flint, readying me for the journey ahead.

Tough times do one of two things: They make us bitter, or they make us better. I'm just crazy enough to believe that everything that happens in life was meant to bring me into the fullness of my original intent. Each hardship makes me less selfish and more aware of what is going on around me. I want to have a word at the ready for those God places in my path that are facing their own kind of hell.

That's the advantage of adversity: It makes way for opportunity. We become stronger, with a capacity to not only walk through difficulties in our own lives but to be a source of help and strength in other lives as well. We become kinder, more compassionate human beings loving those around us with a depth and fierceness that is uncommon, and does not come easily.

I love what my friend Patrick Kitely says about hard places we experience: "Adversity is God's university to add a verse to me."

One of the verses that has been added to me: "We know that all things work together for the good of those who love God; those who are called according to His purpose." *(Romans 8:28)*

May you find your unique opportunity in whatever challenge you are facing today. Blessings & love.

-Raydeane

CHAPTER 4

Rainbow in the Dark

"So we fix our eyes not on what is seen, but on what is unseen, since what is seen is temporary, but what is unseen is eternal." *(2 Corinthians 4:18)*

If you read my first book, you know I love heavy metal music. My favorite musician, Ronnie James Dio, died in May 2010 of stomach cancer. Once again, cancer stole something precious from us – in this case, taking away the best voice this genre of music ever had or will, in my opinion. From 1983 to this day, his music is alive and powerful and still nearly all I listen to.

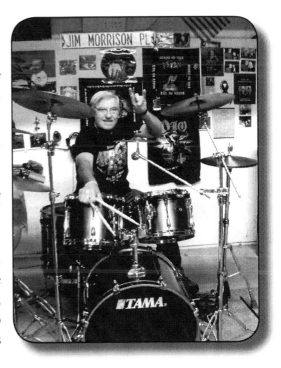

Oh, how we need good metal back. I miss you, Ronnie!

I love to play the drums. When I take the throne behind my Tama drum kit, I rock it hard and loud to my favorite Dio songs. As

Ronnie would say, "metal will never die." I wear a black-and-red wrist band every day in his memory that reads: RIP Ronnie James Dio.

Back in the late 1980s and early '90s, RJD was hated by youth group leaders, churches and parents who were convinced he stood for evil. Certainly, his music spoke of a battle between the dark and the light. But I interpreted it in a different way. I drew parallels to my favorite book, the Bible, where Jesus spoke of angels and demons, evil and divine, Heaven and Hell, the darkness and light "The light shines in the darkness, but the darkness has not understood it." *(John 1:5)*

I want you to know, my friend, there is a real spiritual war going on. Unseen? Yes. Intense? You bet! Can you feel it?

"In the beginning God created the heavens and the earth, darkness was over the surface of the deep. And God said, 'Let there be light,' and there was light. God saw that the light was good, and he separated the light from the darkness." *(Genesis 1:1-4)* Light and darkness is how this world began, and Heaven or Hell is how it ends.

Cancer amplified this war for my soul like nothing else in my life. Cancer is evil and life is divine. From my experience with evil, you better have light to focus on to keep the darkness out of your mind or it will swallow you up.

KID IN A CANDY STORE

In March 2014, at the historic Avalon in Hollywood, California, I had the honor of meeting Ronnie's wife, Wendy. She had invited me to attend the third annual awards gala benefiting the Ronnie James Dio Stand Up and Shout Cancer Fund.

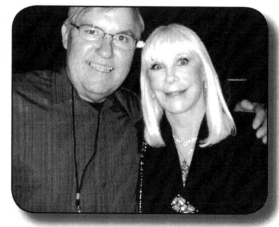

I was able to donate a number of my books to the silent auction to help raise funds for research. At that event, I was blown away to spend an evening with the musicians who played with Ronnie over the years. I actually sat at the table with the two drummers, and sharing words with Vinny and Simon was crazy. The live music was outstanding. It was an evening I will never forget – and know this: without cancer in my life, this blessing would not have happened.

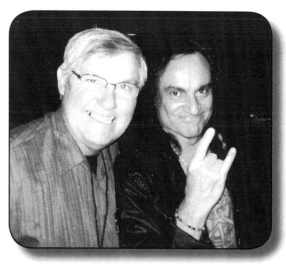

I received written permission from Wendy to use not only the song title but the words to one of my all-time favorite songs, "Rainbow in the Dark." I have listened to this song an untold number of times since 1983.

When I was struck with cancer, this song took on a whole new meaning. There are so many reasons that cancer is my rainbow in the dark. A rainbow reminds us all how precious life is, glowing and bright for all to see for a time, and then gone as fast as it appeared.

And through God's grace, I have found that at the end of that rainbow there is a treasure. For some reason, I have been allowed

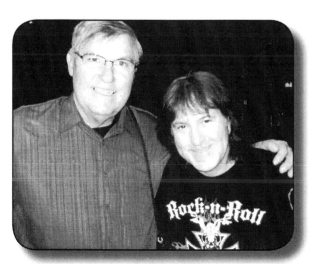

to witness it all, and now to share it with you. I pray it helps you my fellow cancer warrior, or anyone who is hurting, to see the light in the dark of your circumstances.

MY RAINBOW IN THE DARK

The words to Ronnie's song "Rainbow in the Dark" bring back many not-so-good memories from my cancer fight:

Look out
There's no sight of the morning coming
There's no sight of the day
You've been left on your own
Like a rainbow
Like a rainbow in the dark, yeah
You're a rainbow in the dark
Just a rainbow in the dark
No sign of the morning
You're a rainbow in the dark

Cancer warrior, do you feel all alone? I sure did! I was diagnosed with terminal stage 4 lung cancer. There is no stage 5! I was abandoned and helpless in the darkness cast by cancer's storm cloud. My rainbow appeared when all hope for a future was gone, lying on a stiff hard ICU bed with a sentence of death hovering over me. Through the tears of a broken heart, flowing from a broken man, I saw light. Not the light in my room, but light in my heart and mind; in fact, the very Light of the World.

The closer I drew to this light and continued to focus on it, the brighter it became. I began to look at my problem in the light of God's power instead of looking at God in the shadow of my problem. In this light, I realized "hope to cope" – and you can, too.

MY RAINBOW IN THE LIGHT

Back in 2005, Sandi and I were thankful I was still alive. We were no way close to being out of the woods, and my doctors were hopeful but very cautious. Spending time together with family at home was so much better than the ICU. Frail and fatigued, I spent a lot of time in my recliner, legs up and grateful. Some days were pretty bleak, yet I never allowed myself to stay in that sadness. That's why you must have goals and dreams. One long look at Kym's wedding picture would get me through to another sunrise.

One gorgeous day, I asked Sandi if she would drive me to our city park, where a narrow trail winds up a hillside to a special place I call my "God rock." Concerned about my walking ability, she questioned my sanity.

"We need to get to the rock, San," I begged. "I feel today is the day."

Reluctantly, she agreed to hike. Slow and steady with my wood cane in hand, we traversed the trail and arrived at the rock. We looked down at the Spokane River and took in the sights and sounds of God's creation. From this peaceful perch, I had previously seen fish, ducks, marmots, geese, deer and bald eagles. That day the river was roaring and the water was high and turbulent. Even from our rock, we could feel its spray on our faces.

And then, there it was.

Suddenly, Sandi and I were surrounded by the most colorful, magnificent and all-encompassing display of a rainbow I've ever seen. In utmost awe, fascinated by its beauty, we sat speechless, enjoying what I believe was a sign from God. A shimmering wall of colors rose from the river's surface and up over our heads, spanning the panorama of the river below. The feeling was indescribable.

And just like that it was gone.

I believe it's no coincidence that we witnessed a moment like this. When you are invited into God's plan for your life, things happen so you do not grow weary and lose heart and faith. What doesn't kill you should make you appreciate God's grace. This new rainbow in my life confirmed again the shadow of God's hand that covers us.

As long as I live, I will never forget our rainbow in 2005. That cloudless, sunny day rainbow has been in my inner vision ever since, proving that nothing is impossible.

Warrior Words – Kriss

I will start my story from the point where I left a church that I absolutely loved. My family was one of the founding families in that church and I had faithfully attended there for 15 years. I was highly involved... it was my life. Circumstances came about where I had to make the decision to leave the church. I left the meeting with one of the pastors, tears rolling down my cheeks. I closed the church door for the final time and got in my car. As I began to sob, I sat there for a few minutes, turned the key and pulled out of the parking lot. As I was driving down the street, I heard a voice say, "Okay Kriss, now who are you?"

Everything I stood for was wrapped up in that church. That was the beginning of a road to find identity. I realize now everything was working together to direct me into the career field I was created for. There was no option to quit so I fell back on what I knew to be true... that there is always a way through.

My husband worked as a long-haul truck driver. One Monday in September 2001, he called me from Los Angeles and said he had a toothache and asked me to make an appointment with the dentist the following week so he could get it looked at. When he got into town, he told me that he had made good time so he was going to stay home over the weekend instead of driving on to Montana. That was good news since he didn't get home more than once every four or five weeks.

On Sunday, he was out cleaning the truck, climbing in and out, up and down for most of the morning. When he came into the house, he asked me to get him a cup of coffee as he walked into the living room and sat down in his easy chair. A few minutes later, I brought him the coffee and he was sitting in the chair totally motionless. In that short period of time, he had experienced a massive stroke and would never be the same.

In those few minutes, our lives had changed completely. I didn't have a steady job that could be counted on, since I was an intern at a counseling ministry and this happened two weeks after 9/11. His income stopped at that point and life would never be the same for either one of us.

Our relationship changed, our living arrangement changed... everything changed. As I look back on it, I see how God took care of him and what a blessing that was. He wasn't out driving on the Interstate and he didn't have the stroke while he was in the cab of the truck. He was in his easy chair, safe and close to someone who could call 911 immediately.

He spent three months in the hospital and six months in a rehabilitation facility before he could come home with no speech and paralyzed on his right side. He needed 24-hour care. I didn't know what to do, but I knew I had to do something. There was no giving up. I knew there was a way through this and if I just kept my eyes and ears open, I would find a way.

Each day, I had to focus on what was in front of me and get through what was on my plate for that day. I couldn't look to the left or to the right; I couldn't look at anything else other than what I had to do for the day. If I did, it was too overwhelming. There was no option to quit or to let life get ahead of me. I knew we both had to get through this.

Many miracles happened during that time, one of them being that I was able to finish my internship and was hired as a full-time counselor. Even though my income was not supposed to continue, it did. Additionally, for the first time in my life, checks came in the mail that were totally unexpected. People came into my life that provided just the right help at just the right time. Opportunities arose that we were able to take advantage of. We made it through.

Six years later, the ministry where I was employed decided that they needed to downsize so I was let go... in December. With no professional credentials, there was no way for me to get a job as a counselor. So I decided to create my own job. I found an office, created a business structure and was in business by the end of the year (three weeks).

I decided that I needed to get the credentials to be a professional counselor, so I was able to get into a Masters program at the University of Idaho and spent the next two years completing that program and going on to get my professional counseling license. I consistently followed the steps I knew to do to build the business, and slowly but surely, it happened. Did I have doubts at times? Sure, who wouldn't! But in my heart, I knew it would work eventually – it had to. There was no other option.

By 2009, it became apparent that my father (he and my family shared a home) was declining into dementia. So there was a point where I was working, building a business, overseeing and participating in my husband's care at home and looking after my father and his affairs.

Once again, I knew there was a way to deal with all of it; I just needed to figure it out. In that mindset, you have to look for timing and opportunity. If you realize that answers come in the proper time and in different opportunities, you can find a way. We did.

I was able to complete my doctorate in natural health during that time, which filled a need for my father and husband. For both of them, it was pretty clear that medical science didn't have all the answers and that I needed to participate in both their lives from a healthcare standpoint. Dad was sensitive to medication and my husband needed ways to support his physical health because he was wheelchair bound.

I was the voice for both of them and I needed to know what I was talking about because we still had to navigate through the medical world. Having the knowledge that came through that degree helped me to be able to give them both a quality of life that they may not have had for as long as they did. Because the only program available to me at the time was rehabilitation counseling, I not only was able to get my mental health counseling credentials, but knowledge for how to work with disabled individuals was priceless as I moved into the caregiver position with my family members. I did not plan it that way, but I just looked for the opportunities that were available at the time and moved on them.

In 2012 my father passed away. I had never quite understood why my business never functioned at capacity in those years, because I knew it should have, but a week before my father passed, my schedule filled and has been full ever since. At that point I understood that if I had had a full practice I never would have been able to take care of my loved ones the way they needed. It's about timing and opportunity.

Adding the additional education to my tool box widened my scope of practice so that I can now work with my clients not only from a mental health perspective but also from a natural health perspective. That was an added bonus. As I looked back, I realized that I had been given precious time to be the caregiver for both my husband and my father. It was a precious gift. It was a blessing that I was able to have time with my father at the end of his life which not many people get. My husband has also been able to have a quality of life at home that not a lot of individuals in his condition can have.

Even though life has been difficult, it has made me who I am today. I have found that counseling is not just what I do, it is who I am. Even the time I spent working as a bookkeeper and office manager in my earlier life worked together to give me the skills I need to run my own business.

I have found, now more than ever, that Henry Ford had it right when he said, "Whether you believe you can or you believe you can't, you are right." Attitude is everything.

I used to describe myself as a backslidden little Baptist girl who was trying to save herself from the mess she had gotten into and brought everybody in her life with her. That's still kind of true. As a result, because I didn't quit, I have the experience and wisdom to stand at the intersection and point people in the right direction.

Did I have a good attitude all the time? Absolutely not. Did I get tired and frustrated at times? Yes, and sometimes I still do. Did I make mistakes along the way? Sure. Have I learned invaluable things that I can use to help other people? You bet! And that is what makes it all worthwhile.

The point is... never give up. If you do, the game is over. When you are in the midst of difficulty, often you can't see what is really happening and where that difficulty is taking you. If I had given up, I would never have found out who I am and what my purpose is in this life. That information is priceless.

–Kriss

CHAPTER 5
The Tools of a Warrior

For years, I carried a work belt around my waist. The pouch was full of the tools to fix or replace air conditioning and heating units. I needed that assortment of tools every day to accomplish my goals and finish the job at hand.

What if I'd climbed the extension ladder to the roof without my work belt? What could I have accomplished without tools?

Warriors, cancer is a job, and I suggest you show up every morning fully prepared and on time for work. Remember, "A wise man will make tools of what comes to mind." You will need your tools to be a survivor.

There is never a guarantee in cancer, except that it can kill. I do not expect you to become a survivor vicariously simply by my experience. But let me tell you what I know. My cancer-fighting tools were hard-earned in the biggest struggle of my life. They are now priceless to this gray-haired retired heating guy, who got in a fight with stage 4 lung cancer and won. As I share the tools I carry today, you are welcome to strap on the belt, buckle up and choose the tools of a warrior.

Here are the tools I used to fight – and beat – cancer. They all start with F, so I like to call them my new "F words."

MESSAGES IN A RAINBOW: ALL COLORS - FAITH

What is faith? It is the confident assurance that what we hope for is going to happen. It is the evidence of things we cannot yet see. My faith is in no one other than the Lord Jesus Christ!

I share this word first because it must be engaged immediately, right after you're told it's impossible. Faith believes in the impossible. Today, it is not popular to believe in "traditional" faith. That's why this cancer SURVIVOR does.

The Bible says that lack of faith brings many troubles. It also tells us a lack of faith does not invite miracles. And remember, faith doesn't always exempt us from suffering.

Without faith you have no "hope to cope." Listen up warrior, or anyone struggling; faith is being willing to engage with your unseen hope, which makes you able to overcome anything. The darkness will overcome you if no faith is applied to stop it. Like the rainbow, faith is all that separates the darkness from the light.

From my experience, your faith had better be in someone stronger and tougher than your cancer or surrounding circumstances. If not, during the hard times that cancer and life WILL bring, you'll begin to doubt, grow weary and begin fighting blindly. Warriors, we must fight the good fight of faith with our eyes open. Only by finishing the fight do you receive the prize, and that is accomplished only because by faith you stand firm.

Adversity destroys counterfeit faith. We must have faith regardless of the circumstances. (Daniel 3:16-18) True faith grows when it is exercised. It involves endurance to the end, opens the door to new resources and, most important to me, must be demonstrated in our lives.

Is there faith without substance? Is faith reality? I walk by faith and deal with everyday reality.

Dear warrior, I want you to know you must think seriously about faith. It's an attitude of expectation and God can rekindle even the smallest amount. What we can see is just a tiny percentage of what is possible. O you of little faith, as long as a tiny spark remains, a fire can be rekindled and fanned into a roaring blaze. If you feel that only a spark of faith remains in you, ask God to use it to rekindle a blazing fire of commitment to him. I believe that by faith a band of survivors will come forth. AMEN!

BLUE - FAMILY

I have a wonderful family, and I know without their love and support, I would not be here.

As my family grows, when all the in-laws, outlaws, grandkids and everybody else shows up to a birthday party now, we are truly a clan or a tribe.

Do you know family is one of God's greatest resources? He makes it clear we should not take our family's spiritual well-being for granted. Family is so important to Him that He invites us all to join his.

Our nation's strength and our families' strength are related. It's sad but true: family fragmentation may be the biggest domestic problem facing this country. As modern-day society is quickly discovering, there is no substitute for a solid and stable home life. Children without the family tool will probably not learn to cope with the world in a healthy way.

Our families can be a source of both joy and sorrow. Some members are evil, some divine; a family is where love and sin coexist. Why are some of the most bitter fights between two people who married for love? How can people who are so familiar with each other sometimes find themselves so far apart? Of course, things were not intended to be that way. In the beginning God instituted the traditional family when he created Adam and Eve and they became one.

Yet, even in this fallen world, God desires His best for the family structure, and His word holds our greatest hope for the restoration of family.

Family, like faith, will come under severe attack by cancer. I needed my family tool every day during my cancer fight. I have thanked God thousands of times for my family. The sacrifice they made for my survival was incredible. Their love and support motivated me to fight the devil of cancer so I could return to them the same. I was sick with despair knowing I might leave my family. My wife cried for days, telling God she didn't know how to be a widow at 50. My children felt so cheated that cancer could take their dad.

Family was a true measure to see the effect I had on those around me. You can say and think what you want about yourself, but when the rubber meets the road your true colors will shine. The rainbow I witnessed shed light on the truth. I learned gold can't buy the lessons that cancer can teach you.

Sincerity and truth are so rare anymore. Yet when we opened the Morrison family pot of gold at the rainbow's end, that's exactly what we found inside.

GREEN - FACILITIES

I'm convinced one of the keys to my survival was I had the best facilities and the greatest team of doctors and nurses available, period. I believed in them with all my heart and trusted them with my life.

What are facilities? For me this included my cancer center, hospital, doctor's office, nurses, infusion room, gift shop, X-ray and lab, elevator, pharmacy, PET and CT room, cafeteria, social worker, drinking fountain, receptionist, nurse assistants, hallways to walk and the coffee stand.

I want to include hospice under facilities. These folks are great. I thank God I have yet to need their services, but so many very dear warrior friends of mine have spent their last days in their wonderful, compassionate facilities. I thank you for caring, and for being there to assist with all the needs cancer requires. You made life bearable for this warrior and his hurting family and friends.

When you mention Idaho, many people think of potatoes. Living here in North Idaho, we're better known for pine trees, and the only potatoes I see are the ones in the produce section at the local market. Sometimes when I'm raking my yard, however, I wish pine cones were edible!

North Idaho is not known worldwide for its medical facilities. But that is changing. I still dream of a cancer-only hospital, with its own emergency room and everything in one place under one roof. Impossible? Nothing is! Check out the Ohio State University Comprehensive Cancer Center.

Nevertheless, this is home and this is where I was diagnosed with stage 4 lung cancer. I am happy to say our hospital and foundation here have accomplished amazing things in the last 20 years. Kootenai Health is now a member of the Mayo Clinic Care Network, which is outstanding. I personally give the staff and facilities at Kootenai Health and Kootenai Clinic Cancer Services a very big THANK YOU for being part of my survivorship.

Facilities vary from region to region. My point here is not to recommend or condemn, but to make you aware, my warrior friend, just how important those facilities really are. When my incredible oncologist, Dr. Haluk Tezcan, introduced himself to me and my family, I learned he was on call that weekend. That's how we met. Was it fate? I thank God!

I was blessed with this outstanding doctor who continually encouraged me while being raw and straightforward. He never candy coated anything and was very clear with my diagnosis. He was always ready for whatever cancer threw his way. And he knew I was ready and willing to fight. I was willing to work harder and endure more, to reach unseen goals for the prize we both wanted. We fed off our trust in each other. For a broken finger, that might not be so important. For cancer, it's everything.

He was always one step ahead of my 1,000 questions and was just a phone call away. He met all my family's concerns one at a time as we tackled the impossible. How very important this is. Your life and future may depend on it.

If you have confidence in your doctor, like I did, your relationship will become much more than patient/doctor. Well aware I am a man of faith, he would challenge me. For instance, after fighting this battle with him as my corner man for over three years, when the time came to have my port removed, I balked at the idea.

"What if I need it again?" I asked.

He responded, "Jim, where is your faith?"

OUCH!

Our relationship is strong to this day. As I write this on January 1, 2016, I am humbled by the fact that it's now been twelve years since we met. In May, Dr. Tezcan will be the guest speaker at my community cancer group. That's a miracle, folks!

I am so very grateful for my favorite nurses, Peggy, Patricia and Jennifer, along with Sandi's guardian angel Dr. Sarkis, and my rock star Dr. Burnett. Thanks also to Dr. Susan and Dr. York. These outstanding men and women fought hard for me, while well aware of the goals I had set, against all odds: a wedding, graduation and meeting grandkids. In return we won the prize, and now we all rejoice.

I always remind Dr. Tezcan how big a role he played in helping me survive. In his humility, he always responds, "Jim, you did all the work."

I love him for that. I told his wife once, "please don't take this wrong, but I love your husband more than you do." I asked him to write the foreword in my first book, and here is what he wrote: "I thoroughly enjoyed reading this book. I recommend it for everybody, whether a cancer survivor, a patient with a chronic illness, their family, friends or physicians. I do not think this is a recipe or should be read as such on how to survive cancer. Instead, I see it as a story that exemplifies wisdom, strength, values and determination that we, human beings, have. With hope and adaptation, we have a chance to overcome many adversities like my dear friend Jim did." - Haluk Tezcan, MD

I can't stress enough how so very important it is to have confidence in your oncologist and facilities. It's a must!

Don't be afraid to ask questions. So many warriors and their families I meet are not really sure what's going on or what's in the future. Let me repeat: ASK QUESTIONS!

Take control of the fight of your life. At best, warrior, we have one shot to get it right. Don't mess it up for fear of being annoying to those who matter most. I have found they will attend to you based on how you treat them. The professional staff in most cancer centers are wonderful. They deal with desperate people every day, God bless them. They have a calling to help you – and they will! Don't ever hesitate to question anything. We are not dealing with a common cold here. And honestly, time is not on our side.

Look hard at your facilities. Then, decide to give them your all, your trust and your life, or get the hell out of there and find new facilities. Do you want to be a statistic or a survivor?

PINK - FEAR AND FOCUS

Cancer is fear: An emotion of dread or alarm caused by danger. For us cancer warriors fear has a double meaning. Fear can be a profound reverence and awe toward God or a horrifying emotion. I have experienced both. The Bible tells us that if we fear the Lord our God, we will not fear the terror of night. *(Psalm 91:5)*

I fear my cancer, but I am not afraid of it. Does that make sense? When I was notified I had six months to live, fear overwhelmed me and my family. I can think of no other word that strikes fear into someone like CANCER. Our culture equates cancer with death. I know many who, merely out of fear of contracting cancer, have stopped smoking and chewing, changed their diets, exercised like crazy and have even moved to a different part of the country. Are they running although nothing is chasing them?

Is cancer really our worst fear? What about when you send your child out the door for the long walk to school? Or drop them off at daycare? Board the plane for your overseas flight? Maybe the police officer pulls into your driveway with some news you are not prepared for. We now live in a culture full of fear. I believe we have set ourselves up. *(Daniel 5:23)* But I know God did not give us a spirit of fear. So from where does fear come?

When I was diagnosed I remember saying, "My biggest fear has come upon me."

Cancer has been a wrecking ball in my family. Its evil has caused much loss and sorrow. On the other hand, so many good and divine lessons have been bestowed upon me and my loved ones, all from that same evil. How could that be?

Fear wants to become your identity. It wants to dominate and control you. Focus on fear long enough and there is no more hope to cope. Warrior, don't allow fear to steal your future. You bet cancer is scary as hell, but don't allow the fear of it to freeze your faith. By the time it thaws, it might be too late. Know who you are, know what you want and then go out and get it.

I set many goals in front of me, all in fear of my cancer… and all seemingly impossible to obtain. If I had allowed fear to alter those goals, I would have missed so many very precious moments over the last 12 years.

Dio had a song titled, "Stay Out of My Mind," certainly good advice when it comes to the fear of cancer. Instead of the fear, focus on things you can control. I can tell you that a strong focus on the positive eats fear for lunch. Stay focused and sharp. Finish your fight!

PURPLE - FRUSTRATION AND FATIGUE

There has never been anything in my life more frustrating or tiring as cancer. Frustration prevents us from carrying out a purpose. It can defeat us, block us and bring us to nothing. Early in my cancer fight, never a day passed without frustration. Even the simplest tasks became so maddening. Along with cancer, free of charge, comes an 18-wheeler filled with unwanted frustration: At eating, family, socks, God, bathroom, doorbell, wife, failure, church, medical costs, telephone, sex, facilities, pets, doctors, insurance, children, focus, shopping, vomiting and even what's on TV.

Just having cancer sucks; but really, does it have to screw up my whole life?

My biggest frustration? Being told my test results would not be ready for days or weeks. *Oh my GOD!* how maddening that is.

"Scanxiety" is the most frustrating, nerve-racking, sick-to-the-stomach and mind-destroying game ever played. At times, I found even chemo to be easier than waiting for scans and test results that held my fate. Sleepless nights, too anxious to eat, unable to concentrate, yelling at everyone around me and my mind in endless loops…

"What if?!"

"How can it take so long?"

"I'm calling again right now!"

"I don't give a damn anymore."

"I just can't stand it. I need to know right now!"

Come on, cancer warrior, can you give me an AMEN?

If, God help us, I was ever elected president, the very first new law passed would be, CANCER WARRIORS WOULD RECEIVE TEST RESULTS IMMEDIATELY. No more waiting around screwing with our minds. It was so very frustrating to work my butt off between infusions, just to wait and see if anything improved. I could handle immediate bad news better than good news that took a week or longer to hear.

If you are to become a survivor your journey leads through frustration and fatigue. Through a decade of talking with and visiting many cancer warriors, caregivers and others who were struggling, what frustrates me now is those who choose to quit.

Two warriors I know have committed suicide rather than fight on through these frustrations. Bless their hearts; I know how difficult it is to survive. Still, I want everyone to be a hero of hope. I wish all warriors were survivors, but that is just a fantasy. Even with faith and hope in your tool belt, you may ultimately lose the battle. But you can still win the unseen fight.

There is hope beyond the frustrations and fatigue of the here and now.

Before cancer, I was extremely healthy. A common cold would frustrate me to no end. After cancer, those previously simple things became so daunting. Time changed and sometimes it took me all day to get nothing done. Even the littlest project was glorified by fatigue. A very dear cancer warrior friend of mine told me once, "Jim, there is no tired like chemo tired." And he's right. There were many times during my three-year bout with chemotherapy that I could barely raise a fork to my mouth, put socks on my feet or simply even pee. It's hard to focus on the future when you can't even chew or taste your food today.

One day stands out in particular. Just released from the hospital, I was told to rest and stay off my feet. *Hey, that's easy enough, right?* I was at my daughter Kym's house draped onto her living room couch trying to watch TV. The problem started when I dropped the remote. *Now really, how difficult can that be?* With my arm fully extended, the remote was still out of reach. I would have to get up, attempt a retrieve and return to the couch sometime that day. *Should I just ask Kym to help me? No way – I got this!*

Reaching out again with my head extended way off the couch, I started to see stars. *Those damn blood thinners!* I gained my bearings, but realized that the doorbell was now ringing. *Ok, no problem, I can get the remote and answer the door with a two-for-one move.*

The longer it took me to react, the louder and more annoyingly the bell rang. *If I can ever get over there, I will kick their tail.* Finally, with blanket off, I struggled to sit up. Preparing for takeoff, I realized I could not bend over to put my slippers on. It seemed like the volume on the TV and the doorbell went up 100 percent while I was simply trying to stand. *Why am I so beat from just laying around all day?*

The next thing I remember is a paramedic calling my name. Kym had called 911. She said I'd taken one step before passing out and falling hard on her wood floor. She is a nurse and still couldn't handle the situation I put her in. I was so frustrated, embarrassed and fatigued, but I added a new tool at Kym's that day: Tough times never last, but tough people do.

RED - FAILURE AND FUN

Do you give yourself freedom to fail? To fall short, fade away, disappoint?

Back when I operated my own business, I knew a fellow business owner who acted as my mentor. George had started his entrepreneurship at age 12 and had never worked for anyone but himself. He was wealthy and full of business wisdom, and I would pick his brain about my business issues.

I was sure George couldn't even spell failure. He'd say, "I never lose. Either I win or I learn." One day, to my surprise, he told me something that became another tool in my work pouch.

"One of the secrets of successful business people is failure," George said. "They know for every major enterprise that is successful, scores of others have failed. Yet they are willing to risk failure, over and over if necessary, in order to find the winning combination. This is in complete contrast to people who will try nothing unless it seems to be a sure thing."

He went on sharing: "Jim, do you know that your ultimate success will be preceded by an incredible string of failures? But from every failure you will have learned something. That knowledge will eventually teach you not only what not to do, but also what to do to achieve your goal."

I remember the day my oncologist informed me of my first discouraging reoccurrence. I had failed to accomplish anything after a lot of chemotherapy. How could this be? I felt acutely that I had disappointed my family and I began to doubt. *What if I can't beat this thing?*

My conversation with George, years before I was diagnosed, played huge in my mind. Not merely for the success of my company, but for my success over cancer. Failure became my trigger to shoot more faith into being a survivor. I had no choice other than to start chemo treatments again and fight like hell. Death meant failure to me, and I had "made up my mind" that was not an option. A warrior must be a dreamer who refuses to give up.

Failure simply means you're being strengthened not weakened. Please remember warriors, God's work is not limited by human failure. Don't give failure the benefit of doubt. Recognizing your failure is a tool that will ultimately help you succeed – because it causes you to not depend on yourself.

Your chances for success improve with every day you fight to stay alive. New treatments and targeted therapies are expanding at a crazy rate. Thank God!

As a cancer survivor, I have decided to trade in failure, frustration, fear and fatigue and I'm now focused on fun. Yes, fun! *Jim, how in the heck can you associate fun with cancer?*

Well, I'm living it! After cancer, even the little things are more fun. Standing up is fun, and putting on slippers and answering doorbells is a good time. And chasing every sunrise and sunset is way too much fun. Out of my way, cancer!

ORANGE - FINISH THE FIGHT

I've always taught my kids, "pick your fights." What do you do when the fight picks you, instead? *How do I finish a fight I wanted nothing to do with in the first place? Why do I have to fight?*

Our final tool in the rainbow bag is to finish: bring to completion, to actively oppose or combat, as with weapons; to gain by struggle.

I am not a fighter by nature and I never got into fistfights at school. I did have a tremendous number of fights over my dad's drinking, most of them verbal. Sadly, the only fights I ever had in which I had to defend myself were with my dad. With family, those are fights that go on for a lifetime.

For me, the battles in my head are the toughest. Unseen, they are thoughts fueled by my selfish desires. On the playground in my mind, they distract me from my good fight of faith. As Ronnie would sing, *"LOOK OUT!"*

We live under the curse of a fallen world. After eating the fruit, Adam and Eve, who had previously known only good, now came to know evil. Today, darkness and light are in constant battle. Whether you believe it or not, there is a spiritual war going on all around us at every moment.

We cannot dismiss the Bible's teaching about angels and demons as nothing but myths from the past. Especially when we live in a culture with an increasingly secular worldview. Evil and divine are in the center ring warring for the final foothold of mankind, a fight fought with unseen weapons in the arena of your mind.

We know how cancer attacks our physical being, but it's just as important to pay attention to the way it attacks our mind. Cancer is infamous for its mind games, and I believe our mind can be our weakest point. Sometimes our tools and weapons are too physical. We focus too much on what we can see, touch, read, taste, hear and smell.

I realize that cancer is viewed as Goliath, a fearful foe, unbeaten and invincible. Yet David won that fight by using a non-traditional weapon. What motivated that young shepherd boy to take on the impossible?

To finish this fight for our lives, we need purpose and discipline, along with an array of weapons, both seen and unseen. My most important weapons are a positive mindset, a set of impossible goals and the faith to witness them coming true. I urge you, don't fight Goliath with the world's usual and useless weapons. Don't go in alone!

Your fight, my friend, will lead you to experience things you never knew existed. You will walk by faith into places you have never known before. You will witness the darkest of darkness but can also witness the Light of the World. When the rainbow appears in your darkest moment, you'll know why.

Here's my advice, my brave warrior. Don't worry about armor and a sword. A very small stone and the courage to fight the giant will do just fine.

CHAPTER 6

Caregivers Are the Real Survivors

"Courage does not always roar. Sometimes courage is that quiet voice at the end of the day saying, I will try again tomorrow."
– Mary Anne Radmacher

We cancer warriors receive all the attention, but without our caregivers we would not be here. My caregivers paid a hefty price for me to wear that survivor's band around my wrist. While the warrior carries the heavy load of defeating cancer, their precious caregiver carries all the loads. Along with the rest of life's burdens, they must face their warrior's cancer, along with their own fears and changes in routine. Overcoming cancer is the only big job the warrior faces, but for the caregiver, cancer becomes another overwhelming demand out of many. It's truly a team effort.

KEEP CALM AND HAVE A PLAN

At every book signing, speaking engagement or visits with fellow warriors and caregivers, I make it a point to express how absolutely important it is NOT TO PANIC. I have met with a number of families who, simply because a CT scan was required, are already running without anything chasing them yet. Don't do that!

Of all the survivors of cancer I have been honored to meet over the past twelve years, one trait sets them apart: They all led their teams with a surprising method of self-control in the out-of-control world of cancer.

Our culture loves flashy and flamboyant, yet if you are to be a successful team in surviving cancer, you will accomplish your goal with steady hands and sober minds. Trust me!

People don't study cancer in preparation of receiving a diagnosis someday. None of us ever think it will happen to us because cancer is something that happens to other people, right? Wrong! I never smoked, so I figured I wouldn't have to deal with lung cancer. Only recently, the FDA acknowledged that, "smoking is not the only risk factor for lung cancer."

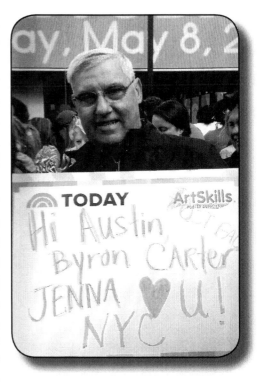

Sandi and I are well aware how hard it can be to avoid absolute panic, especially after the cancer storm strikes and you realize it's just ripped the roof off your family's life and your house is taking on water, fast.

From my experience with cancer, I believe there is no cookie-cutter approach to taking on this foe. One size fits all does not work in the cancer world. Every cancer, chemo or radiation has its own side effects, both physically and mentally. Everybody handles the pain and sickness differently. I have met men and women who, bless their hearts, can't, won't and don't handle any of it in spite of their team's request to fight on.

One day I took one of many visits to the oncology floor at our hospital. I was there because a friend had shared my book with a new cancer patient's family and they'd asked me to visit. I was greeted with hugs and "Thank you so much for coming."

The warrior's family suggested we leave his room and go into the hallway so we could talk freely. I hate when this comes up because I already know what the problem is. The family told me, "We love him and are here to support him, fight with him and for him, we want to be his team."

They continued, "But, he can't handle having cancer or the extreme pain he's now experiencing. He says repeatedly that he will not do any chemo. He just wants to die, rather than fight. We all feel so helpless."

"How old is he?" I asked

"He turned 59 last month."

"And how long has he been in the hospital?"

"This is only day two," they admitted.

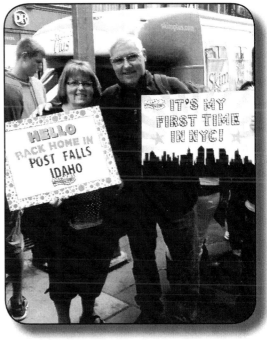

I am sad to tell you that this fellow warrior died on day nine. Life passed as fast as the storm that took it.

Believe me, after what I've been through, I understand perfectly well why someone would want to throw in the towel. My point in sharing this true story is to help you understand that the battle is real for every family, team and warrior. There is no right plan; we all must fight and earn survivorship, or not, on our own.

The key is to team up with fighters. If you falter, your team will enter the ring for you, ready to fight their fight and yours too. God bless our caregivers.

DO YOU REALLY WANT TO SURVIVE?

"Jim, I want to be a survivor."

Sooner or later, on my first or second visit with another warrior,

I hear this plaintive request. I caution them with a strange question: "Are you sure you want to be cancer survivors?" They usually look at me as if to say, "Of course, you goofball, why even ask that?"

There are so many events and crazy things to deal with. Certain decisions at the right time are critical, along with staying on date for infusions even when your blood pressure is through the roof. Not being able to eat or just not wanting to, then getting your ass chewed for losing weight. Yelling at your caregiver over whether to take this pill or that, while the school calls to say that your 2nd grade grandkid fell off the monkey bars.

Oh good, now the caregiver has something to do and that gets them away from me. HA HA.

I think this guy named Murphy had cancer, because if it can go wrong it does. To survive this mess, you and your team are in for the battle of your life.

Of course to be survivors is the ultimate goal. But, those words are just too easy to say without knowing how much it will cost both you and your caregiver to earn the right to wear that name tag.

Growing up, I spent a lot of time with my mom's dad, who I nicknamed Paw. A hard-working Italian, he was full of old-school common sense. You may not know what common sense is, because it's not common anymore.

Paw taught me years ago, "Jimmy, if you can't find a job, make one." I followed that advice. Not finding a job that could pay what I needed, I made my own. I started my heating and air conditioning company from scratch with an old Ford truck, a ladder, a work belt full of tools and a prayer.

Trying my best to prepare for what my dream envisioned ahead, I had no idea of the cost involved with becoming a successful business owner. My mentor, George, would remind me often, "Jim, you don't own your business, it owns you." After many days of long hours and things out of my control, and much learning of cash flow, taxes and the like, the business and I survived – and thrived. The company is even more successful today, thanks to the team of my brother-in-law caregiver, Gary and his breast cancer warrior survivor wife, Julie. AMEN!

Knowing now what it takes, would I start another business? Yes! I love the challenge. I love being the underdog, being told there's no way, you're crazy, the percentages are against you to be successful. I especially like to hear that something is impossible.

My new impossible job is to be a successful stage 4 lung cancer survivor. This job found me, by no choice of my own. I unwillingly accept the position. With asbestos exposure early in my career, we now have a major problem, Houston! I never imagined that working in the field I loved would expose me to a killer. My cancer diagnosis was the toughest challenge I've ever encountered. Yet, we survived.

Yes Jim, we want to be survivors regardless of the cost. Then you will be!

For you see, to survive may not mean that cancer doesn't kill one of your team. To me, survivors means you fought the good fight, it will not be easy or comfortable. It won't be painless; being a survivor does not guarantee the absence of struggle and the abundance of strength. Often it means great cost and sacrifice with no earthly merits. Being a surviving team will cost you friendships, jobs, some family members, leisure time and treasured hobbies.

But while the cost of survivorship is high, the value of doing it together is even higher. Survivorship is an investment that lasts for eternity and yields incredible rewards. Whatever happens during your fight with cancer, you can now move on without regret or doubt knowing you gave all. You fought the good fight; and gave it your best.

I admire you. Your team inspires my caregiver and I to encourage others with this evil disease to team up and fight on. So they, too, can be survivors. God bless you all!

THANK GOD I HAVE CANCER?

I am so blessed to be alive and to be able to enjoy the elementary school performances of my grandsons, Byron and Carter. No matter what's going on with my cancer schedule, I make time to be there. Kids spell love, T-I-M–E. As the saying goes, "Make time now, or you'll find time to regret later."

Before a recent performance, Sandi and I took our seats in the crowded auditorium, spotted our beloved Carter Sauce and waved our encouragement. I noticed a young lady in the front row of children who kept her head down. As her third grade class took the stage, she raised her head and enthusiastically sang. Wow, what passion and excitement she brought to that part of the program. Concerned, I asked Carter afterwards if he knew who I was asking about.

"Oh yeah, Papa, I know Emily, she is fun to hang around with."

"Why does she look different to me and why doesn't she look up until she sings?" I asked.

"Papa, she has no eyes."

Two years ago, I felt a need for our local communities to have a cancer group. Along with some handpicked fellow cancer warriors, I started a Warriors of Hope cancer wellness group. These meetings have really taken off and are a great place to share stories: good, bad and ugly. Cancer has its own language; and you really need to be talking to mentors who speak it.

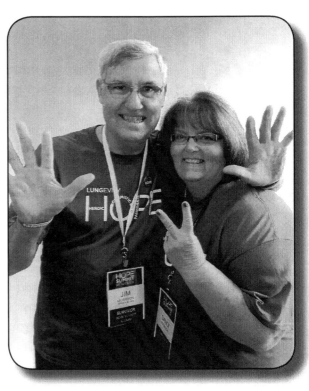

I was at our library to sign in for the meeting room for Warriors of Hope. A woman behind me said, "Excuse me, sir, are you a cancer survivor? I noticed all your bracelets."

"Yes, I am!"

"Do you lead the Warriors of Hope?" she asked.

"Yes I do, we meet every month on Thursday here, and you are welcome to attend."

"Well, my name is Carol, and I lead the Alzheimer's group here at the library every Wednesday. It's so very nice to meet you. I've heard about the good work your groups achieve."

"Well, thank you Carol."

"Jim, I would love to lead a cancer group."

It sounded odd to me.

"Why would you say that?" I asked. Her response floored me.

"Oh Jim, I would much rather lead cancer groups because you guys have survivors."

A longtime friend told me that his mom recently passed away from Alzheimer's. He shared how over time everything got worse and worse. And then he said, "Jim, I'm so grateful for one thing Alzheimer's could not take from Mom – and that was her prayers. I would sit next to her and listen to her pray, and Jim, the prayers she would put out to God, beautiful powerful prayers. That evil disease stole everything from mom but her ability to pray. It was the only thing she remembered." Oh, how the prayer of a righteous warrior is powerful and effective.

No one needs to tell me what cancer is capable of doing. I have heard and seen it all after 144 months of being in the foxholes with my fellow warriors. And I still carry much collateral damage from frontline encounters. I must say, at times, I find us warriors to be whiners, complainers and crybabies – including ME. Cancer is not fair, and why we have been chosen beats the heck out of me. But complaining has no place in cancer camp, in my opinion.

I have been humbled again *(Daniel 4:37)* to realize that many others have it way worse than I do. This morning I witnessed another sunrise. Do you have eyes to see? Then look forward through the windshield, not backward in the rearview mirror. Focus the eyes you have on your unseen goals, and always remember warriors and caregivers of cancer. Though few overall, we have the capability to become survivors. It is possible. I am one!

For some, that will never be an option. When my time runs out,

I will sit with my friend's dear mother and listen to her pray, with eyes that can see why she never forgot how.

The Bible says that life is too short no matter how many years we live.

Let's quit whining and finish the fight!

Yes, THANK GOD, I HAVE CANCER!

QUESTIONS I PONDER

Bless those who are the caregivers; those who put their own lives on hold to help us warriors survive. My entire team devoted themselves to my fight. But did my experience with cancer change my wife too? Did she witness the same rainbow I did?

To be honest, Sandi and I have different views on our cancer battle. Sometimes in the heat of the fight, I just assumed she was reading the same book I was. Not so! But regardless of our different approaches, we shared much along the way. During the most desperate times we would wear our pajamas all day and just cry and talk and cry some more. We called them our "crybaby" days. This time spent together was powerful. It brought healing and renewal as we shared our true feelings and drew strength from each other.

I suggest every team we mentor have crybaby days. My only caution: DO NOT STAY THERE! On tomorrow's sunrise, restart your fight to survivorship.

It's also the right time to get your personal belongings organized. Having a will, family trust and funeral arrangements are NOT a sign of weakness or failure. I planned my funeral service with Sandi on a "crybaby" day, and so should you. It's very important to handle this stuff. If someone on your team thinks by doing these things you're giving up and quitting, bench them or trade them! Team Survivor must be truthful with everyone involved. Cancer is not a mere game to be played, nor is it politically correct. If you handle it like that, it will win.

Sandi's biggest fear was being a widow at 50. I did not want to bring the thing she feared most upon her. With that thought continually on my mind, I believed it helped me stay focused. It was in the fourth year of our battle, when I was declared NED, that I realized God answered Sandi's prayer when her husband survived.

Throughout my fight with cancer, I cannot honestly say that was the most pressing goal I thought about. Sure, I love Sandi immensely. We have now been married 44 years, since high school, and that's an incredible run. I will always be in debt to her caregiver skills. But sometimes we are not on the same page in the warrior's journal.

Sandi struggles sometimes with the amount of time I don't spend with her. Our crybaby days are long gone. She cannot understand at times why I am so obsessed with writing books, signing books, meeting warriors, speaking engagements, e-mails and phone calls. She has mentioned to me more than once, "Jim, you are all or nothing." I will admit much time and effort goes into being a warrior of hope. I try to explain to Sandi that my battle's not over.

I cannot be content knowing I survived cancer and that's it.

I know survivors for whom the opposite is true. They feel that the cancer part of their life is behind them and they are going to live life to the fullest, do what they want and go where they want. They tell me they want to enjoy their life in the time they have left and never look back, go 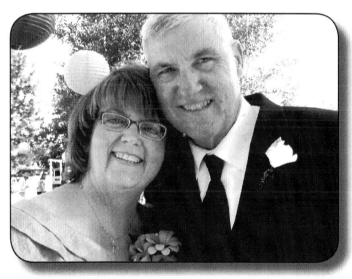 back or discuss what they been through.

I believe the Lord extended my life to be a living example for others to observe that doctors don't know everything, odds don't matter and statistics are just numbers. I am a challenge to the evil of cancer; it wants to control the amount of light my fellow warriors see. But by faith, I say *GO BACK TO HELL!*

Cancer still tries its evil best to find ways to uproot our relationship and cause chaos between Sandi and me, allowing diversion and doubt. Since we both survived together, why wouldn't she understand my burden to help others? What happened to me that didn't to her? We have discussed this in depth, and I believe we agree on the answer.

The difference was my rainbow in the dark, something I alone experienced in that hospital room. God answered my prayers and breathed into my heart from the Book of Daniel. At that moment, I understood without a doubt that God is in complete control. *(Daniel 5:23)*

Not only did God deliver joy, hope, peace, and life for a humble heating guy and his high school sweetheart, but during that most desperate, darkest time in our marriage, he also set us apart to offer light to those who don't know what he is capable of.

Sandi pours her entire life into children. Her dedication, especially to her grandchildren, is unmatched. Our new little Jenna is under Sandi's watchful loving eye three full days a week, her job by choice.

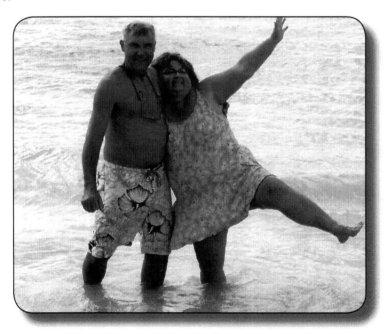

If she's not there, you will find Sandi volunteering at school where our older grandsons attend. She volunteers hours of her now-free time, and I support her dedication and love.

For me, my extended life is for others to read, ponder and hopefully glimpse what the Light of the World can accomplish in the darkness of cancer and life.

By faith in God, we praise Him for precious life together and overcoming evil. I pray for you my fellow warriors, caregivers and all who struggle. Are you sure you want to be a survivor? If the answer is truly yes, then you and your team will give it your all.

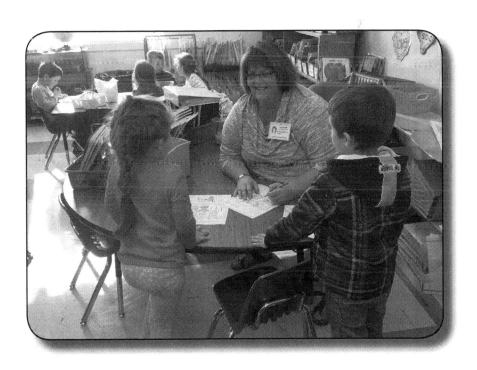

Warrior Words – Kim

At the time of my diagnosis, I was 42 years old. I am a wife and mother of four children. Three words I thought I would never hear in my lifetime… You have cancer! Not only do I have cancer, but I have the deadliest kind of cancer: Stage 3B adenocarcinoma non-small cell lung cancer which spread to my lymph nodes. Only a 10 percent chance for a five-year survival rate. How could I have lung cancer? Isn't that a smoking disease? We were blindsided and extremely scared by this news.

Frankly, I was pissed off! I did all the right things and was good to my body and I get this??? I had absolutely no symptoms. Now I was faced with two options…One, give up and let this disease win. Or two, fight like hell because I refuse to let my family see me suffer from this disease in self-pity. Don't get me wrong, I have my crybaby days. But the key is not to stay there because fighting this disease will consume you physically and emotionally.

I am currently in remission for two years. It hasn't been easy getting here. July 1, 2013, I went in for a routine CT guided biopsy of my lung. Ha! Routine procedure my butt! can you hear the sarcasm in my voice? It went horribly wrong. I got an air embolism that traveled to the chamber of my heart and gave me a heart attack. I coded on the table! I died! They tried to revive me for 20 minutes. After seven broken ribs I woke up. It was not my time to go!

If this didn't kill me, surely cancer couldn't. See I'm a fighter! As my dear friend and mentor Jim Morrison would say… finish the fight! I am so grateful for his help along my journey. I was doing 37 radiation treatments and simultaneously doing chemotherapy once a week every three weeks for eight months. I've had five thoracentesis and one pericardial infusion which I had drained. I tolerated chemotherapy pretty well. Of course I prepared myself for the worst.

There were days I couldn't get out of my recliner. I recall a day where I was so physically exhausted I couldn't move another step and sat down on the kitchen floor for a couple of hours. That was pretty much a low point in my life sitting in the dark on the floor by myself crying because I couldn't muster the will or the strength to stand up.

As strange as this sounds, losing all my hair was the hardest part! Good thing I don't have a bumpy head.

I am so grateful for my faith and family. Without them I'm not sure I'd be where I am today! My sweet husband, Dwight, has never missed a single doctor's appointment of mine. This is really tough on him. He lost his mother to this awful disease 13 years ago and now his wife is facing the same situation. I'm on a gene targeting chemo pill that I take twice a day.

The fear of cancer coming back is real! I get "scanxiety" every three months. I know I'll have to fight through some bad days to earn the best days ahead. I DON'T HAVE AN EXPIRATION DATE! I will continue to fight to see my kids grow up and to see them have babies. God bless.

–Kim

CHAPTER 7

To See Another Sunrise

Why is it that the sun rises on both the evil and divine? Does it not rise on the mass shooter and the church pastor? Does it not rise on loving parents as well as those who abort their children? Does it not rise on our traditional American flag and the rainbow rag? Is it not the same sun?

Our human nature assumes that no matter what we do, evil or good, the sun will rise. So we carry on!

Have you given any thought to a sunrise?

Do you pay attention to the beautiful eastern skyline on a crisp, crystal-clear early morning, as the sun breaks over the horizon? Do you view in awe its fresh colors that explode light over us all? Do we even think about tomorrow's sunrise?

Cancer makes you appreciate that sunrise!

Rising and setting day after day since we were born, that sun has become just another mundane event within this culture, like marriage, church, family and all old-time traditional things. They don't have the same meaning anymore.

Have you ever given any thought to who makes the sun rise? There's some force out there controlling its movement. How else on one very special day, could it stop shining and allow total darkness to cover the entire earth at three o'clock in the afternoon?

TO SEE ANOTHER SUNRISE...

Look familiar? This is the title of book one. I wish I could share all the emails and letters from the people who read it. In fact, many people have told me they bought the book because of the beautiful sunrise on the cover.

Jim, how can a sunrise help me? I have been in darkness for so long that I can't bear to see the light of day.

Welcome to the club. I was there myself. My answer for you, my friend, is one single word – *HOPE!*

For years now, I have been witnessing impossible sunrises and chasing every glorious sunset. To me, the sun's rise and fall have been renewed into the sacred event the creator meant them to be since the beginning of light.

Why is this event such a big honking deal to me? Because cancer stole my business, some of my health, and three years of my time.

Yet cancer's evil is no match for a rising sun. A cloudy day is no match for a sunny disposition or a sunrise. From dusk to dawn, darkness thinks it rules, but light will kick its butt every time! The darkness of evil and the evil of cancer never will overcome or extinguish God's light. AMEN!

God used an ordinary, everyday thing that we usually take for granted, a sunrise, to give me new hope. My early goal when odds were impossible was simply TO SEE ANOTHER SUNRISE. A new day meant winning another round over cancer. Focusing on the colors of hope within the rainbow in the darkness enabled me and my family through our battle with cancer. From that fight, which my team finished, we cherish not only every sunset, but our marriages, our children, grandchildren, our church home, every breath we are allowed and our precious lives.

Sandi and I still go to bed each night with the hope TO SEE ANOTHER SUNRISE and even if we don't, we rest in contentment and peace. *(Daniel 3:16-18)*

This morning, the only thing that rivals another sunrise is this beautiful little baby granddaughter walking, jumping and laughing around our living room, softly saying, Papa, Papa. Jenna is such a precious miracle. My fellow warriors, and anyone else who finds little meaning and hope in life anymore, do you realize the excitement it means to beat the odds and be part of Jenna's life?

I encourage you to take the hope that comes with every new sunrise and make it personal. Tomorrow's sunrise is for you. Claim it and chase it. Don't waste a single day! Count it as a blessing bestowed on you by the grace of He who is unseen.

LIFE IS TOO PRECIOUS

Don't doubt and delay any longer. Don't allow mundane, joyless days to discourage you. Hey, if anyone could have done that, it was me, when I was given only two hours to live. Remember, I'm a cancer guy. I want you to know I despised lying in bed all day every day. No way, I told myself, I would get dressed and go to my chair. I lived in my recliner for three years, and in that chair I spent a lot of uninterrupted time, reading, thinking and hoping.

Some days all I could do was watch TV for hours. If you have health challenges you know the days I'm talking about. But I learned something from all that nonsense on TV.

I learned today's world is full of pain and bitterness. People feel deep disappointment, overcome by life's storms that blow in and wreck havoc. They find themselves buried with problems that defy solutions. There's a high tide of discord, distrust and disharmony sweeping across this country. Most people have a feeling of their own futility. They are so busy with the real struggles of everyday existence they didn't even notice today's sunrise. Can hope be effective anymore?

I never realized how many pills and medicines are available now to help us "cope without hope." Just ask your doctor, and bingo, you're good to go – that is, if all the side effects don't kill you.

Have you ever seen a news headline or commercial offer hope, instead of thrills and pills, to make you feel better? Perhaps we are over-thinking our ills. How did my grandparents and parents ever survive without all this stuff we have today? I bet it was hope; that sense of how precious a new sunrise and all of life really is.

TO SEE ANOTHER DAY OF HOPE

From scripture, hope means a strong and confident expectation. By its very nature, hope deals with things we can't see or haven't received. Hope, like a sunrise, renews every day. It's your choice to live by hope or exist in despair.

But let me warn you, side effects do exist with hope:

Hope changes how we see ourselves.

Hope changes what we value and what has meaning.

Hope affects what we do with our lives, talents, time and treasures. Hope gives us joy and peace.

Hope gives us protection, strength, courage and boldness.

Attention fellow warriors and caregivers! Hope gives us endurance, comfort, and confidence in the face of death.

God intends to let the world know that there is hope beyond the problems of the here and now. The signs of hope outshine all previous disasters. As you consider this, please look hard at the prospects for your future, cancer and all. I encourage you to lay hold of God's promise of rainbows and hope.

LOOKING FORWARD

Hope is an unseen weapon, just like most of the other tools I used to survive. Unseen weapons not only change your chances but they change your character itself. The rewards won with unseen weapons, like faith and hope, are of infinite value. That's why, although people don't always understand me, I can say I'm thankful for having had cancer.

Those unseen weapons are seen by those around you who witness your actions and accomplished goals. Family, coworkers and fellow warriors see the results of faith and hope. They hear the results, and follow those with their own faith and hope. Our example is more powerful than any drug on TV. We offer the real thing.

I was invited to speak at a Susan G. Komen survivor's event at the beautiful Coeur d'Alene Resort. My family was there in full attendance. Closing my talk, I walked over to Stephanie and kidnapped my little Jenna. Holding her high and proud, this is what I said:

"Warriors, caregivers and survivors, this beautiful baby held in my arms is what *hope* looks like. She is what *faith* looks like. I love this goal I hold."

People in their desperate place need serious weapons, not the crap this world offers like false hope, pills and prestige. Those things provide no help in the darkness and desperation of

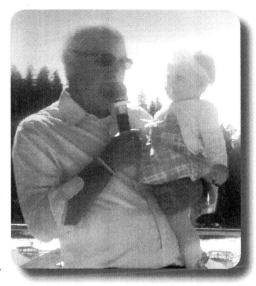

a life-threatening disease. How much money is needed to guarantee you're a survivor of anything?

Stretched out in my recliner chair, reading my Bible on a miserable day four after my chemotherapy infusion, I read, "For everything that was written in the past was written to teach us, so that through endurance and the encouragement of the scriptures we might have hope" (Romans 15:4).

With Daniel and those three young men, I followed their plan and watched their actions. I didn't see anything on TV in three years as powerful as the unseen tools these men had on their belts. It told me if you are without Christ, you are without God and without hope.

Hope is God's fuel to get you through the darkness of cancer or anything else. You must believe and have hope in hope and your unseen weapons.

Hope is what empowered me to see another sunrise – to look forward, not back. Instead of asking, "Why me?" I changed my thinking to say, "Why NOT me?" I found I could wake every morning to a new day fresh with hope, even on day four of chemotherapy.

Another thing I discovered about hope is it cannot be shattered or altered. Like my "battle buddy" Steve in book one. Every day I visited him he was looking out his sixth floor window for that helicopter to deliver his new heart. He never gave up hope though he

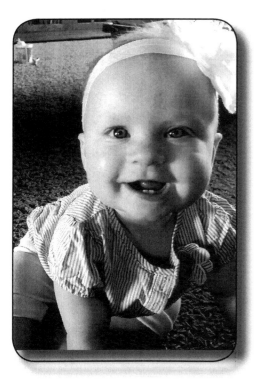

waited three months. Please keep hoping. You never know which sunrise brings with it your new heart. What if Steve had given up on hope, and quit his fight the night before?

I learned from Steve. I fell asleep and awoke every morning with the hope that today's sunrise would bring with it my remission. Many sunrises and sunsets passed and I never gave up that hope. I just filled my tank again and again.

I remember one particular morning, before going to the cancer center, sitting with my legs up in my recliner, feeling the hope that today's sunrise might be the one to freedom. As we waited for Dr. Tezcan to enter the exam room, Sandi and I held onto that hope. Oh, the wonderful words he shared, as this sunrise delivered the wonderful news I had waited a year and a half to hear: "Jim, I am confident you are in remission."

Incredible! My heart swelled with emotions. I wondered – without the true hope that comes only from God, could I have waited 18 months for my first remission?

No warrior escapes by his or her own great strength. But if we hope for what we do not yet have, we wait for it patiently. May the God of hope fill you with all joy and peace as you trust in him, so that you may overflow with hope.

May the force - of HOPE - be with you!

Warrior Words – The Harpers

My 45-year-old husband of 25 years was given two weeks to live and our world was instantly rocked! We had two choices to make: give in to fear, or find the little glimmer of hope inside us and fight. We had recently received a prophecy at our church, speaking about the big plans God had for my husband. We had peace because we chose to believe that God wasn't through with him yet. The day he got his leukemia diagnosis, he told me that he had perfect peace and that this was truly the best day of his life. He knew where he was going if he died, and he knew that if God wanted him to live then he wouldn't be in this fight alone. From the beginning, his true faith inspired us all. He had his occasional moments of doubt, when he wished for a guarantee that he would be alive for his children's graduations, weddings and future grandchildren. There were thousands of people praying for him. One of our friends drove 13 hours through the night just to pray for him in person and anoint him with oil.

"Is anyone among you sick? He should call in the church elders and they should pray over him, anointing him with oil in the Lord's name. And the prayer of faith will save him who is sick, and the Lord will restore him; and if he has committed sins, he will be forgiven." *(James 5:14 15)*

This is not to say that Chris didn't suffer, struggle and go to "hell and back." As our pastor puts it, "he was jacked up!" He had numerous complications and setbacks along the journey but we kept pressing on. His attitude was unbelievably positive. He had decided that this was out of his control (not easy for a Type A former marine) that he needed to trust God and "let God" carry him.

We learned in a hurry to take each day one day at a time. We listened to praise and worship music literally 24 hours a day. We focused on the good things and we became so grateful. I know it sounds crazy, but every day we found something to be grateful for. Sometimes it was just that the day was over. Another thing we did as a family (we have four children ages 12-20 at time of cancer diagnosis) was to laugh a lot and try to find the humor around us. Believe it or not, if you're looking for it, there are many funny things that happen during cancer treatment. Quite a few of them revolve around bodily functions.

He had seven week-long, hospitalized chemotherapy treatments, along with additional chemotherapy, total body radiation and a bone marrow transplant. Thankfully there was a selfless donor out there so now my husband has life! Now that he is "normal" (we are supposed to call it our new normal), cancer seems like a distant memory. Here are some qualities we have acquired since our cancer journey: patience, love, faith, hope, trust, a tight-knit family, gratefulness, compassion, empathy, love in action, perspective, appreciation for each and every sunrise and a deeper spiritual walk.

So would we go back in time and rewrite our story without cancer? No, most definitely not! We know that this was part of God's plan for us. He brought us through it and we would never go back.

-The Harpers

CHAPTER 8
Who's Really the Sickest?

This chapter is raw, harsh and discouraging. It's also deeply personal. I intend it to be so! If the next few pages don't make you shake your head in disbelief, then I have wasted your time and mine.

There is a sickness in our world that rivals the toughest cancer. Our culture no longer uses a moral compass and sacred values are all but gone. Every day I read or hear about another sick story. In my little sphere, these stories hit hard in the stomach and heart.

I was exposed to this culture of deception years ago, when I visited my dad in a halfway house. His vodka addiction had taken over his life. I entered a beat-up, ugly hotel, and after a full pat-down for drugs and weapons, I was allowed upstairs. I stepped over and around men and women sleeping and sitting. I declined several offers of cigarettes and prostitutes.

I knocked my special code on dad's door and walked into his room that was smelly and messy, full of cigarette smoke and lit by a single bare light bulb. Our discussion was terse, as always. After we ate a couple of TV dinners, for some reason he begged me to stay the night with him. It was a first. Hesitant and fearful, I called Sandi and let her know.

My stay there in hell was a night I will always remember, although it happened 30 years ago. I can still vividly recall the yelling, fighting, smell of weed, police sirens and loud sex sounds. Dad snored comfortably, while I lay awake all night, wondering to myself:

How and why could my dad be so sick?

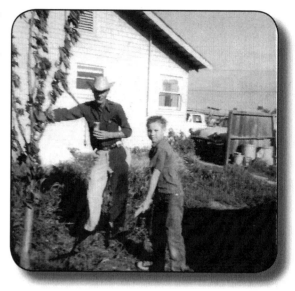

By this point in my life I had been saved, baptized and now served as youth group leader at our church. I knew the Light of the World, but here in my dad's world, nothing but darkness prevailed. I was haunted by questions. *Did he see any light in me, coming from me? Could he tell the difference between divine or evil anymore? Was I really any different myself?*

I needed to go to the bathroom and walked toward it in the dark. I felt something strange under my bare feet. I turned on the light and was horrified to find that the floor was black and moving. I could see my footsteps marked by dead and half-crushed cockroaches.

I did my business and walked back to the dank couch where I was sleeping. I shook the sheets like crazy, but I could still feel the bugs moving on me in my imagination.

But once I'd switched on the light, I realized, those bugs had vanished. They couldn't stand the light. This lesson from long ago is still bright today.

I can tell you that my own previous addiction to porn thrived in darkness. That's where I hid and enjoyed it the most. Only by bringing it into the light, and not hiding anymore, did I receive healing.

Now, after cancer, I am much bolder to flip the light switch on, to see who runs and who does not. What great things can happen if the Creator of Light empowers you and me?

Come on, church! Our culture is sick and blinded by darkness. Ever notice how much light a single candle can throw into total darkness? If we are chosen people, a royal priesthood, a holy nation, a people belonging to God, then let's declare the praises of Him who called us out of that darkness into his wonderful light.

REAL LIFE DOWN AND DIRTY

That day in my dad's awful apartment, I witnessed the nature of hell on earth. I am overjoyed to say that my father did not stay there forever. After my mom's death, he cleaned up his act and found a better

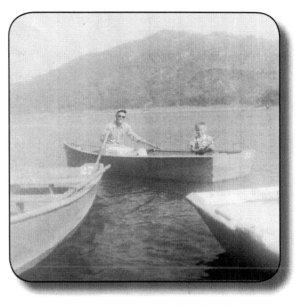

way of life. He reached out to me, and we reconciled before he died.

I do need to relate some ugly, yet true, stories that expose the behind-the-curtain tricks of the wizard of cancer. These are stories I have either witnessed personally, or I know a member of the family in which the event occurred.

I want all caregivers and warriors to be aware, whether Christians or unchurched, male or female. No matter how well off you may be or how strong you think you are, be alert! Don't be caught off guard by the danger that cancer brings to a family or a relationship.

LIKE A JUDAS KISS

One of the most horrifying effects of cancer I've watched is family abandonment. I've seen the people that cancer warriors trusted most give in to their own selfishness and retreat, instead of offering a helping hand in the hour of need.

I watched a husband, right in front of me in the living room of their big beautiful home, as he betrayed his wife, newly diagnosed with breast cancer, and their three small children.

His hateful words still ring in my ears: "I have no time for this. I can't afford to waste my time with cancer. I have a business to run and my time is way too valuable to be babysitting you. Call your lazy mother and put her backside to work. I don't have time for this nonsense."

With inner resolve, I held my fist from swinging toward his ugly face. I knew that without his emotional cancer in her life, she had a better chance to survive.

And survive she has. Five years NED. Bless her warrior heart!

So thank you, lowlife, prideful spouse! You give love a bad name. I thank you, although you would not make a pimple on a good man's ass, for embarrassing me to be a man and thus making me look hard into the mirror. And for freeing my fellow warrior, allowing her and the children to put their faith in someone worthy and dependable instead.

THE RESTROOM FROM HELL

Sandi and I were invited to an American Cancer Society fundraiser in an elegant hotel in Washington State. Although I am honored to be part of these events, I hate the suit and tie stuff – it's way out of my comfort zone. It was a gala evening with great food, and we raised a lot of money for cancer research.

After drinking a lot of coffee and a little wine, I was on the hunt for the nearest men's room. For some reason I had removed my name tag and left it on our table. I located a large restroom. There were two other well-dressed gentlemen inside. They were evidently attending a separate doctor's conference, which I could tell from their conversation. I hadn't seen them at my cancer event, and likewise, they had no idea who I was and that I was a survivor.

As they talked, one doctor told the other something that stopped me cold.

"There will never, ever be a cure for cancer, since there's no profit in a cure."

I tell you what, that doctor was lucky I did not want to ruffle my tie that night. I was absolutely outraged.

I thought of my Tarceva pills that cost me $12,800 a year. My chemotherapy sessions had been $45,000 each. I'd maxed out a million-dollar health plan in a year. *How could a doctor even say such a thing?* True or not, that attitude was from hell itself. I was weak in the knees to hear how far our priorities have fallen.

"In God We Trust" should now read, "One Nation Under Greed." When did money become more important than saving lives? When did money become more important than families? Our goal should be to use all our resources to assure families a long and loving time together, nurturing and teaching their children till death do they part.

That's why the Bible says, "The love of money is the root of all evil." Don't we realize that ill-gotten gain will destroy us faster than cancer ever will? This type of money will eat us from the inside out. Think about it!

Are you a cancer warrior or a caregiver without piles of money, but with pockets stuffed to overflowing with hope, faith, joy and peace, enjoying a rich life each day? Are you looking forward to precious events, seeing another sunrise, a birthday party with family and chasing another sunset? Are you living in total contentment with the unseen treasures received from the pot of gold, which now in your heart are priceless?

Or are you following today's culture, in pursuit of money, but owning absolutely nothing that matters? They worship what they see though blind eyes. They praise the gods of silver and gold, of bronze, iron, wood and stone, which cannot see or hear or understand. What do they have that is priceless?

I believe someday there may be a cure for cancer. Yet right now, I believe without doubt, there is already a cure for sin.

WHERE'S THE BOYFRIEND?

My daughter, Kym, played softball in high school as a pitcher on the all-girls team. Two of her teammates were twins. These girls were a hoot and they spent much time together on and off the diamond.

When I was diagnosed, these twin girls helped Kym through some pretty rough times. Sandi and I had the privilege to watch these young girls grow up. Their parents were faithful fans and attended every game, home or away, like we did. Spending this amount of time each season, we became fast friends. One day, Sandi and I were informed that the twins' dad had been killed in a motorcycle accident. It was a sad and tragic time, and the girls needed support. We helped as we could. At this time, I was NED for three years, and my oncologists felt pretty confident we had accomplished the impossible.

I would run into one of the twins occasionally at the gas station, grocery store or bank. It was always great seeing them, hugging them and hoping to run into each other again soon. The girls were well aware of the book I wrote in 2012 about my cancer journey, and they were very supportive.

Kym called me and asked if I was sitting down. That's never good! She said, "Dad, the twins just found out their mom has stage 4 cancer, and they would like you to sign a book and visit their mom."

Of course I would! We discussed the heaviness of cancer, talked through her personal affairs, and asked how she was set up for medical and money for the future. She shared her late husband had held a substantial amount of life insurance. She felt she needed to go to Arizona for treatment instead of using our local facilities. She told me, "I have more confidence there than here." I was sad to see her leave. She was aware stage 4 is tough, and knew full well she could run out of time before she gained victory. I did my best to prepare her for the fight for life.

After she arrived and got settled in, we stayed in touch weekly, sometimes daily. She was proceeding nicely and getting into "rhythm" with the chemo. After three or four months, that point when chemo really started taking its toll, I stopped hearing from her. Concerned with how the twins were handling this, I checked in with them.

They told me, "Mom has a boyfriend now. We haven't met him yet, but he looks clean-cut and seems good for her."

Keep in mind, this gal was all alone 1,500 miles from family and friends. I questioned whether the boyfriend was such a good thing. I had a bad feeling due to past experiences. Cancer can cause people to do the wrong thing. How many false fundraisers have you heard about, with people using cancer for personal gain? Money is the root of all evil, cancer is evil and evil attracts evil people. Look out!

I tried to reach her every day with no success. Finally, after relentless pursuit, I got her on the phone. She gave me a lengthy tirade against cancer, the facility and chemotherapy. "It's not fair – why me?" she kept asking.

I understood her anger and hurt. I was glad she felt safe enough to vent and share all of her true struggles with me.

"Jim, don't be concerned about my boyfriend," she said. "He's only here to help me. He really is a kind, loving guy. He treats me like the Queen of Sheba. Every day he is faithful coming in. He likes and enjoys serving my needs, brings me gifts and gets anything I want. He will be answering the phone, handling my personal business and such and just keeping an ear and eye on everything. Thank you, Jim, for calling, I promise I will do my best on this end. I'm doing better; it's tough, but I'm tough."

"Yes you are, girl," I told her. "I will be calling often, you can bet on that, I promise!"

From that day on, every phone call was intercepted by "the boyfriend." I was interrogated about who I was, how I knew her, whether I was family, and exactly why and what I was calling about. It got to the point where I believe he was watching phone numbers and began choosing who could and couldn't talk with her. Guess which list I was on?

An old trick my business mentor taught me, when it was time to collect the bills, was to call using another phone number. As soon as they hear your voice, they know you outsmarted their little plan. I collected a ton of delinquent bills by doing this. Now that I knew when and where they were, the next time they heard my sweet voice, I was standing in their office or on their porch, with the game over.

My plan worked enough times, using enough different numbers, that soon the phone lines became totally silent. I could not talk with her even going through the cancer center's nurse station. I was tempted many times to hop a plane and walk into her room. With all communication gone, she was off the radar.

Many months later at her funeral, Sandi and were invited to sit by the twins. A respectful crowd of family and friends were gathered to pay respect to the tough "motorcycle mama" she was. It was a moving and fitting service, done well in her loving memory.

During the service, I kept scanning every face for the boyfriend. Where was he?

I tried my best to be respectful and not embarrass Sandi like I most often do when it comes to cancer work. I took the twins aside and asked where the boyfriend was. The girls were broken and hurt, hugging me and crying on my shoulder. I tried to offer words of hope and compassion. I know what it feels like to lose your mom to cancer.

It was like they knew. I'm not sure how they sensed it in me, but out of the blue, one twin said, "Jim, thank you so very much for bringing comfort to our mom. She would always say to us how you encouraged her and put a smile on her face when you called. I know what's bugging you."

"What is that?" I asked the lonely twin.

"That boyfriend stayed around to help only until the money was gone," she said sadly.

I ask you: *Who's really the sickest?*

WHY THE DARK BASEMENT?

I have met with fellow warriors of anything, anywhere. It does not matter to me where and what, as long as if by God's power I can help. There is one place I really hate going into, and that's the VA hospital. I really have a tough time in this place, and my heart goes out to the men and women who put their lives on the front line for me and my family. They grant us freedom and the home of the brave, by risking their lives for our wonderful country.

I know a local pastor, J.O., who is very supportive in helping cancer warriors. His wife is a three-time survivor. He understands the ongoing battle and how it hinders your hope and future. In fact, they opened their church as the first venue for the community cancer group that fellow warriors and I hold once a month.

One day, J.O. called to ask if I could visit a man with a very bad cancer diagnosis.

"Jim, he's a tough one," he said.

"What do you mean by that, J.O.?"

"Well, I visited him today, and he threw me out of his room, so I thought I'd call you. You can handle him and I can't."

"Thanks a lot, dude, for throwing me to the lions."

"I'm serious, Jim, he really needs to hear your story, and more importantly, your faith. He has a hard time with 'preachers' as he called me. Can you please go for me? He's in the cancer ward."

"Hey, J.O., which hospital?"

"Veteran's," came the reply.

My heart sank. I'd been excited for the challenge until I heard what a hellhole this real-life warrior, and now warrior of cancer, was held captive in. This place drains me and sucks the winds of hope and faith right out of my sails. I considered calling J.O. back to tell him I just couldn't make it.

But then I made up my mind. *God, cover my back, I'm going in!*

Our VA hospital is far from my home. It takes way too much driving time for me, and by the time I arrived my mind was all screwed up. I kept thinking about all the hurting, but hoping-to-see-another-birthday cancer sufferers I had visited in here, both men and women, and sadly I realized that not one of them had survived. *Is that right?*

The cancer ward was located in the basement. *Really, the basement?* Some of the patient rooms were old converted janitorial closets. It was dark, depressing and everything else cancer brings to your mind. I really struggled here, to the point of being sick from the smell of decay and abandonment. I continue to this day to thank God, over and over, for the facilities I had.

I stood in the doorway to his dimly lit room.

"Hi Edwin, my name is Jim," I said. "May I come in for a short visit? Edwin, I'm a cancer survivor and would like to visit you… Edwin, I won't stay long…"

Nothing but silence.

Then I was rudely greeted with, "GO AWAY! GET THE HELL OUT OF MY ROOM."

Well hello to you, too, I thought. *Screw you and this place, I'm out of here.*

Walking over to the nurse's desk, I asked, "Is Edwin always a complete jerk, or is it just because I'm fresh meat?"

"Let me put it this way," she said. "He's difficult."

I was beginning to see how J.O felt. If the powerful message that God is love was not going to work on this war-torn hard heart, what would?

And yet I persisted. I went back to annoy him once again from the doorway.

As soon as he saw me, he turned his TV up so loud that the nurse was immediately in the room cussing him out.

Then Edwin turned on me full of fury and said, "SON, ARE YOU HARD OF HEARING? I ASKED YOU TO LEAVE ME THE HELL ALONE!"

I swallowed hard, calmed my temper and thought quickly.

"Well, I would, sir," I said. "But your daughter asked me to visit you, sir."

"How do you know my daughter?" He asked belligerently.

"Well sir, I know the preacher at the church she attends, and he discussed my visit with your daughter Jenny, and she approved."

"What does she care?" Edwin spat out. "She don't give a damn about me."

"I beg to differ, sir. By asking for help she is showing that she loves you. She's just not able to show it in here, sir."

"What is your name?" he barked.

"Jim, sir!"

"WHY IN THE HELL DO YOU KEEP CALLING ME SIR?"

"Because I honor you, sir, for what you have done for my freedom, and that of my family and for your outstanding service to this great country, sir."

There was silence. I could see the tears in his eyes, though he tried to hide them behind his pride.

As I finally sat next to his bed, Edwin and I had begun to communicate. I wanted nothing, needed nothing, I prayed for only his time. Our little chat was the subject of much speculation by every nurse on the floor that day, because Edwin "Let someone in!"

I sensed a hurt and broken man who had covered his true feelings for a long time. Edwin's real adversary in that cancer bed was pride. I believe his pride had changed his identity, so much that even his own flesh-and-blood daughter could not get close to his wall or even want to try. In its own way, pride can make us way sicker than cancer ever will. There are survivors of cancer, but pride always leads to total destruction.

Our peaceful visit lasted a half hour until I mentioned the words God, heaven and hell. He loudly proclaimed, "THERE IS NO GOD, HEAVEN OR HELL. IT IS WHAT IT IS AND THEN YOU DIE."

I'm not sure I said or did the right things, but I visited Edwin as best I could, and I hope I gave him a sense that I did care for his outcome. He did eventually throw me out of his room, after I read Daniel 4:37 and asked if I could pray for him.

"YOU WILL NOT PRAY IN MY ROOM!"

On my way out I paused, looking back at him.

"Sir, I hope I have not become your enemy because I told you the truth."

Just as I entered the hallway, I turned and prayed for him.

"DAMMIT JIM, I ASKED YOU NOT TO PRAY IN MY ROOM."

"Sir, I did not pray in your room, I prayed for you sir, from the hallway."

After bowing his head, he looked up into my eyes, with tears again in his, and very gently replied, "Jim, thank you."

He would never allow another visit.

I paused to collect my thoughts, sitting on a bench in dire need of a fresh coat of paint. Instead of going out the easy way, I walked up the stairway onto the main floor. There, veterans lined the hallway. They were playing cards with one arm, sitting on the floor with only one foot or a patch over the missing eye. There were men and women on crutches, canes, some pushing walkers. A lot of the wheelchairs had bent rims and tires wobbling for those with no legs remaining. Some just stared off into the distance. Others were in full conversation with someone I couldn't see.

I couldn't even bear to peek into the rooms. This place was more depressing than any infusion area or converted hotel I had ever been in.

My cancer was a Sunday picnic compared to what these brave souls had seen and been through. I am thankful that my dad, a Navy veteran, never experienced this injustice. I continue to be crushed every damn time I pull up at the entrance to this facility and commit to *"Going back in!"*

When our veterans are hurting, why does this country spend billions of dollars to locate a tree with a monkey in it on Mars? Why do we pay out more money to end life before birth than we do to save lives after? We spend enough money every cycle on political elections to build two new VA hospitals in every major city. I wish that, just once, we could witness what billions of taxpayer dollars could accomplish if our leaders would resolve, make up their mind, for our nation, for us all. What if we spent our money wisely on urgently needed and important things: finding the cure for cancer, creating good paying jobs, giving tools and helping people to function as a traditional family again?

What the heck do we do with that tree on Mars if we do find it? I believe that if God wanted us on Mars, I'd be writing this book from there.

I'd like to see us spend money on something that has life-changing effects here and now; on positive, constructive things that will bring real hope and a future to all lives that matter to God! How about first, let's treat our veterans with respect and offer the health care they deserve.

I am ashamed that a veteran commits suicide every 65 minutes in this country, while the national VA suicide hotline sometimes goes to voicemail or makes callers wait on hold for a long time. I am ashamed that our obsession with pet dogs means they often get better medical care, have more rights, eat better and are loved more than our retired warriors. What have we come to?

I think about Edwin, who died alone in that dark basement, not knowing for certain the God who created him and the country he fought for cared about him deeply.

Who is really the sickest? I invite you to take a deep look at your own priorities, and how you treat others. It's some of the strongest good that can come out of cancer, or any other dark place.

Warrior Words – Dr. David

I just had a chance to read your book that you gave me at the Washington HOPE summit. Thank you for sharing your cancer journey with me and with the world. Very inspiring! And very selfless to share the very personal details of your struggles on many fronts.

You are very lucky to have had a supportive family during your diagnosis and treatment. One thing I did not share during my talk was the fact that when I was diagnosed my wife told me (literally), "Oh well, everyone has to die of something." Then she left me. I thus became solely responsible for our four kids, ranging from 6 to 12 years old and had to deal with working as an academic clinician and single father for the next five years until 2005 when I married my current wife, who has been a dream come true. This was very difficult, but all of us have emerged stronger than ever, with God's help.

Best regards, enjoy your family and your hunting trips, and perhaps we will cross paths in the future!

-Dr. David

CHAPTER 9

Strong and Very Courageous

This chapter is dedicated to fellow cancer warriors whose time ran out, and who have shown strength and courage like no others I have met. I honor my fallen warriors. Cancer is most certainly a war; an unseen fight for our life that sometimes ends with death. War is always a tragic thing that comes with casualties. I could write a whole book on just fallen warriors I have known. I miss them all! Please hang with me – these stories are more positive than you might ever imagine.

For this book, I chose a special three. These great warriors allowed me to become a small part of their fight for life. At a very tough time, some not knowing me from Adam, they frankly discussed personal matters pertaining to life and death, heaven or hell. They have offered their last ticks of time with me to share a sip of water with them and pray.

I love the raw, really deep questions at the right time. I depend on God for the answers, and it heals us both. These strong and courageous folks have given me tools to survive when all seems lost. They have inspired me to inspire them and others in the future. I visited them hoping I could encourage them, when in truth, they encouraged me.

When I consider all these fallen warriors that blessed my life, I really struggle with survivor's guilt. Why me, that I would be set apart to survive? How does God choose when and who and why? For now, by His grace I am spared, and with that thought in my heart I push forward by faith, not looking back.

Believe it or not, the most encouraging people I have met in my life are my fellow cancer warriors. It's true! If you want to offer encouragement, then come across as encouraged. I remember when I was really sick, it was terrible when someone would leave me feeling worse after their visit. Bless their hearts, but they were not on the right page; only God and cancer can enlighten with words that mean something.

Why is it, when cancer is involved, that most people are willing to share God's true word? In the darkness, is there any other that can offer light?

Cancer divides the light from dark and truth from lies. We may never listen or hear the Lord's true words until cancer or a terrible life tragedy softens our heart and gives us ears to hear.

Over my years in church, many brothers and sisters have taken me under their wing to offer mentoring, counseling and accountability. During my fight with cancer, especially in the very beginning, our church was wonderful with help and support. After many years now of wonderful, powerful time spent with people of cancer and their families, I have come to this conclusion: tragedy is where we are often tempted to quit, but in truth, it is where true faith and commitment to God begins. There is no triumph without starting at tragedy.

In fact, our best shot at surviving starts at tragedy and the seemingly impossible. I have been blessed to witness faith and truth in action, miracles and life-changing healing in people and their families. My most recent unbelievable, uplifting spirit-filled days of conquest have been in a hospice room, living room or ICU, not church. *Why is that?* Because when I'm around cancer people, there is no such things as politically correct. There are no hoops to jump through, no dress code, no drama and no qualification for membership. We warriors deal only with the very essentials of life.

I love my warriors who have passed on. These brave souls earned their victory by being strong and courageous. By hope they endured the storms and tribulation of life and the destruction of sin, and they stood firm in the face of evil. They've given so much more than they could ever take. They have mentored me and others around them from their very death beds. Their most amazing trait to me during their tragedy is when they showed incredible empathy for others.

These fearless warriors changed me with their positive attitude and heartfelt words. In this brief life, we meet those who stand above the rest. I believe these people are handpicked to intervene into our lives at the very time God appoints them to do so. I find it reassuring to know that evil is no match for the total control of God.

I have lost count of how many funerals I've attended and performed. I pray, in their honor, I can be the same type of strong and courageous person, so someday someone will remember my influence on their life. From my deadly encounter, I have been allowed by His grace to rise up from tragedy, attend boot camp and now, continue to carry on the fight these brave warriors fought.

They have shown me that those who are fit to die are the most fit to live. Now I have a clear understanding of how precious life is and I know Who holds my hand. *(Daniel 5:23)* I am not afraid of dying anymore, because I already have.

STRONG AND VERY COURAGEOUS

The very first time I met Clint was a cold call. He had no clue I was coming.

His friend had asked me to visit, so I drove to the rehabilitation facility where he was recuperating from a recent surgery.

When I walked into his room, all I found was an empty bed and a can of Pepsi Max and the TV blasting "Duck Dynasty." Looking under the bed, in the bathroom and closet, I asked the nurse his whereabouts.

"Look in the workout room," she said.

Yeah, right, I thought. *From what I hear this guy's been through, there's no way he's in any workout room.*

"Who's Clint?" I asked the nearest person as I peered into the workout room.

Wow! I was already impressed by this guy's courage. There he was, lifting weights, doing leg lifts, sweating and focusing on survival.

From that first visit, I knew I wanted to be around Clint. A number of visits later, Clint would ask me a very important question:

"Jim, are you content with your cancer?"

"Yes Clint, I am."

"How did you reach that point?"

"Well, my friend, one early morning lying on my ICU bed and waiting for the sun to rise, I realized I could not rely upon myself but in Him who raises the dead. Clint, we have not been dealt a hand we understand, nor will our families. I believe you and I have been set apart so that our God can use this time to take two screwed-up boys, and make us into the men and fathers we strive to become."

I recall that every one of Clint's goals, along with every thought and breath, were always about his family. Not once did he ever say, "Boy did I get cheated out of life. Why me?"

I never heard him complain, moan and groan or wallow in self-pity because he had cancer. He did not understand, nor do I, but we were content whatever the circumstances. *Are you?*

One thing that amazed me was his wife, Kelly. I was incredibly touched by her unconditional love, support and never-ending time with Clint, day after day. So I was blown away to discover that they were divorced. Knowing this made her time and love for Clint even more astounding. Kelly had since remarried, and many times in our very sincere and personal conversations, Clint would say, "Jim, I would marry Kelly again in a minute if I could, I love her so." To watch them together, now in a hospice room, floored me. I could feel their passion and concern for each other.

Clint and Kelly had married young, had three daughters together, and even when they split, had done everything with the health and happiness of their daughters foremost in mind.

Clint loved his daughters, and spent time with them at every opportunity, even painting their nails for them – a real act of love from this rough-and-tumble man. Kids spell love, "T-I-M-E" and that's what real men give their children. Thanks to cancer, once again I had met someone who inspired and guided me on my own path to being a real man, who helped me take a hard look in the mirror and raise the bar.

I finally asked Kelly one day, "How does your husband feel about your never-ending time spent with Clint and the girls?"

I was so impressed that I wanted to meet her husband, Kevin, and share my heartfelt respect. He invited me into their home for a conversation. Awkward as it was for me, even after nine years of meeting men involved in cancer warfare, I spoke directly to thank him for his example and witness of how a real man handles himself.

I asked how he could be so understanding and compassionate with Kelly's situation. He said, "When I met Clint's girls for the very first time I knew I was going to marry Kelly." *WOW, would another man think that way about my kids? Would another man find my Sandi attractive by the conduct of our children?*

Men, think about the impact of those words. Do your children reflect the man you are?

Kevin went on to compliment Clint and Kelly for raising wonderful children who showed respect and compassion for others. Kevin told me that his own son was forced to have both kidneys removed at a very early age. This had required 24/7 care, total sacrifice and putting Kevin's own life on hold. That's why and how he knew what she was about to experience with cancer.

I was blessed to be invited into this wonderful family, and blessed by God who extended my life to meet them. Because of my fellow warriors, Clint and Kelly, I will do my best to share this story whenever I can, to restore and hopefully inspire other families, to be real and seek the truth. To be REAL men and women, it is our duty to God and each other to set an example for our children and our society, to share the light given us to lead others out of their darkness. It is

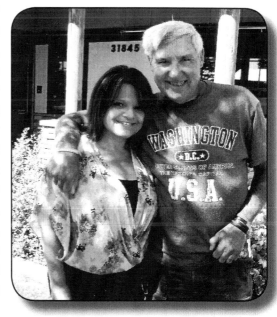

my hope that every person and family may discover, and then put into practice, the blessings awaiting them at the end of their own rainbow in the dark.

So I continued to visit my new friend to encourage him, and instead, Clint encouraged me. I was so impressed by his heart and his attitude. At his house one day, I rang the doorbell and knocked. Clint yelled to me, "I can't turn the doorknob lock, my hands and fingers are so swollen."

He suggested I crawl in through the kitchen window, which I would have done in order to visit him. But he couldn't stand up from his wheelchair to open the window due to his weak and swollen legs. Now frustrated, Clint suggested this time I go to the garage and he would open the garage door.

Standing outside in a snowstorm, I began to wonder why it had been five minutes. Now panicked, I raced from window to window looking for him and calling his name. *Where was Clint?* I heard the garage door going up.

"Sorry Jim, I got over to the opener, stopped and fell asleep in my chair."

Just a simple goal of opening a door, with two grown men, both with a terminal diagnosis, determined to accomplish it. I will treasure our talk that day forever. We shared how God looks down from heaven on the sons of men to see if there are any who understand, any who seek God? Clint read to me Psalms 37, "If the Lord delights in

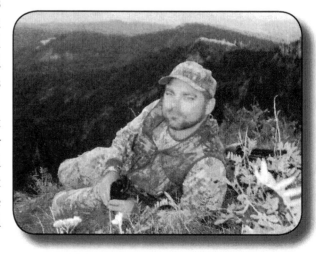

a man's way, he makes his steps firm, though he stumbles, he will not fall, for the Lord upholds him with his hand."

On my last visit at hospice with my fellow warrior, I asked if he was ready to meet the One in whom we trust? Clint assured me he was. Through the tears of a broken heart, I shared with him that God will never let us down. Though His ways are not ours, He is in control of all things. He will sustain us on our sickbed and restore us from our bed of illness.

God's peace is different from the world's peace. True peace is not found in positive thinking, in the absence of conflict or in good feelings. It comes from knowing that God is in control.

I was so honored to perform his funeral and for his family to allow me to share how their loved one helped me through my fight. My warrior Clint had gone home. And now, in his loving memory, I share what he asked me one day to share. "Realizing that life is short helps us use the little time we have more wisely and for eternal good."

In one of our many visits since Clint's service, Kelly told me how the girls had asked for a sign for closure and reassurance as Clint lay dying. That sign came when, at the very moment Clint took his last breath and went to heaven, Kevin walked into his hospice room. The girls ran to Kevin for his love and compassion and to bond with another real man.

God carefully chooses the time when he calls us into his presence. Precious in the sight of the Lord is the death of his saints. Clint was strong and courageous; please honor him by having ears that hear, and faith that matters.

SURVIVING THE TRAGEDIES OF LIFE

Sometimes you just have to learn things the raw, tough way. Thirty years ago my mom was diagnosed with colon cancer. At that time, just one type of chemotherapy was available. And there was very little, if any, relief from the side effects. It was hell and I witnessed my mom suffer. Her suffering made me suffer and thankfully, made me tougher and better equipped for life's tragedies.

When it came my turn, I received four different types of chemotherapy treatments plus pills for nausea, injections for blood counts and waited a year for a new pill to be FDA approved as a targeted therapy. Cancer is still evil and always will be, but research has come a million miles since my dear mother's time.

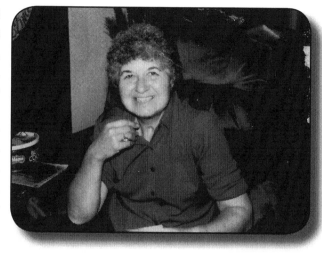

And yet, there is a ton of research left to accomplish. Please fund research – the precious cure is near! If you have lungs, you might need it!

During my mother's illness, I had no clue how to fight, not only cancer, but the tragedies of life. This disturbing event took place at a time I did not know who or what to believe. I was struggling for some sign of normal life. My family was a dysfunctional circus, my dad's drinking problem by his own choice rendered him useless, my kids were young and money tight, my sisters overwhelmed with work and family, so that put me as ringleader. Inexperienced with evil and how harsh life can be, blindsided, weak and powerless, I was absolutely unprepared and challenged like never before in my young life. *Let the lessons begin; may I be man enough to hold up and fight with her.*

My mom's body took tremendous punishment, but I believe it was her mindset that cancer had no punch for. From round one, mom was committed to a course of action. No matter how hard each round was or how many of them, she had children to raise and the gates of hell would not stop her. Her mindset was to witness her children grow up, graduate and get married. And she did! She even met and spent precious time with some of her grandkids. My mom lived way longer than anyone could have predicted. Why? I believe it was her attitude and mindset. She finished the good fight!

Mom lived eighteen months from diagnosis and died at age 56. Her death absolutely crushed me. This is where tragedy tried to end any triumphs in my future. But I learned from mom what it looked and sounded like to be a courageous warrior, and now it is my honor to pass her legacy on to you and others.

In hindsight, after my own experience with the same enemy, I clearly understand how very strong and very courageous my mom was. I miss her so much after all these years. My dad died of lung cancer at 62. Oh, how I would love to share and show them what God has performed in their son's life.

Mom was living with us the last year of her life. My dear caregiver wife treated my mom like her own. Sandi was so compassionate and loving. I know it brought much joy to Mom during a very desperate place in her life. I would spend hours at bedside with her. With no tools of my own at that time, I was at lost for the things to say. Time and touch are so strong when nothing else will do.

She told me about her visions and thoughts. The one she shared the most was about a bright light which drew very close and asked her the one thing she wanted the most. Mom said, "To see my children grow up." The heart of a warrior is focused on others. It's not about you anymore. One of cancer's blessings is how it makes us realize we don't own the rainbow or our life; they are both on loan.

One evening I noticed her bedroom door slightly open and I could hear her talking. Eavesdropping from the hall, I could hear clearly the words she spoke. I was amazed that every word was for the good of others. Not once did she mention her situation or feelings, and not once did she ask for relief from her pain or vomiting. Jesus never prayed a miracle for himself.

There was my sweet mother in a prayer of gratitude, thanking God for Sandi and me for being such a blessing to her and asking for wisdom on how to encourage her family. I noticed during this intrusion into her private time that both her hands were folded together in her lap.

All the while she was praying and talking, her hands were in circular motion, outlining the thumbnail on her left hand with the thumb from her right hand. I never asked about her little ritual. In some way it must have helped her.

During my own battle I, too, had my little talks with myself and the Lord. One nasty day soon after my chemo infusion, I was so very sick and fatigued I could barely sit up, but I did. Struggling to hold myself on the bed's edge, I folded my hands on my lap. To my amazement, I found my own hands in motion, outlining the thumbnail on my left hand with the thumb from my right hand.

Now I knew exactly what Mom was saying in silence with her hands.

ROCKY

His name was Dom, short for Dominic. I call him my little Italian warrior, and he was a pistol indeed. I thank God that my first book brought us together. Our first meeting was at our local Denny's. Two hours later, it was clear that our meeting was not by coincidence.

Dom's personality drew you in and that's what he wanted. He was truly concerned and would help anybody; he treated me like we'd known each other for years. He was old school and the real deal, which is rare these days, but so refreshing. His stories inspired me. During our conversations over coffee, he shared many stories from his youth and career. One stood out in particular. As a warrior, I always listen for attitude: Is it positive or negative? What's truly in your heart is what the mouth speaks.

Dominic told me of bar fights he would look to start, standing all of five foot eight and weighing maybe 170 pounds. His height and stature reminded me of the small but powerful Ronnie James Dio. I questioned why he would do such a stupid thing. Had he been drunk? No!

"Oh Jim, that's what everybody thought," Dom said. "This crazy little Italian calling out the biggest guys in the bar. I would just work 'em up to place bets on how fast they could knock my head off."

"How are you still alive?" I asked the Italian Stallion.

"It all comes down to attitude," Dom told me. "They were only looking at my outer appearance, so they would fight to collect the bets. What they did not realize, until after I collected all the money, was what I had inside."

On my first visit to his home, which turned out to be just five miles up the hill behind my place, I met his equally fiery pistol wife

Patt. She was an outstanding caregiver and great support. Dom had a great teammate.

Dom was a special warrior to me. I was very stable with my cancer at the time we met; I think I was NED about seven years. This guy would light me up with enthusiasm, all while he dealt with a tragic diagnosis of non-smoker stage 4 lung with metastasis and eight months to live.

I spent hours with Dom one-on-one. He really liked to email, so every day he sent something. You develop this crazy warrior's sense of humor. I opened one email with the heading, "Can't afford a real nurse." The picture showed Dom hugging his new, good-looking cardboard cutout nurse. Fun is a great "F" word. Use it, it will help you finish the fight.

Eventually, Sandi started going on the visits with me. Patt needed help with the whole thing too, and Sandi shared much about our battle. Dom was one of the strongest fighters I have been around. He was always doing and trying everything to fight on.

His cancer was relentless; they could never slow it down or contain it. The chemotherapy treatments almost killed him. Strong as he was, his heart just could not handle them. His lungs kept building up fluid, which is something I really struggled with. They installed chest tubes to drain and relieve the pressure and help him breathe. Eventually, he required full-time oxygen. Running out of options, he fought on.

Dom had very good weeks and some very, very bad ones. During his fight for life, he was very concerned for his son and daughter-in-law. Like any marriage, there are always

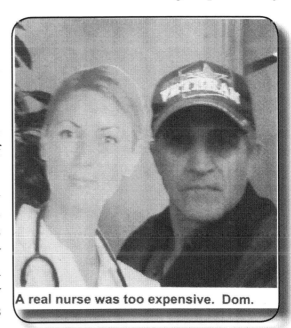

A real nurse was too expensive. Dom.

needs. His son needed leg surgery so had it done at the same time Dom was sick, in order to spend time and bond again with his dad. This time together was priceless to them both.

As a man of prayer, Dom was always praying for someone other than himself. His prayers for me humbled me so. This man was dying and still he prayed for my continued health so I could help others. *Warriors do what warriors do.*

He requested his son to pray every morning and night for his wife and marriage. During Dom's fight, he witnessed his son come to peace with his situation. It was a goal accomplished during the very toughest part of his cancer battle. That goal brought great joy and healing inside, where Dom was the strongest.

Toward the end, my warrior friend was growing weaker by the day. One morning I received an email that made me cry. For the first time I sensed defeat. That's a "D" word and I know it well.

"This cancer has beat me," he wrote. "I quit. I can't go on, and there is no use to fight."

After praying for help, I called him. Patt answered and shared her feelings. I felt that we needed to see them. Sandi knew Patt loved chocolate cake so before our visit we picked up a beautiful cake. When we went to their front porch, we saw a sign that Dom had put up on the door.

The sign read, "TO LIVE TO SEE ANOTHER JIM."

My war mate was sprawled over the couch, frail and weak to the point of not being able to sit up. Barely keeping his eyes open, he welcomed us with slurred words.

I reached my hand out to hold his and he responded with a wink. I bent over and kissed his forehead.

"I'm here for you, my friend," I whispered. "We will get through this."

"Jim, I'm done, I wish I could be like you, you're a superman, a better man than I am. I can't beat it; it's got me, I'm going home."

"Hey Dom, you want some chocolate cake?"

"Look at me, Jim, do you really think I want cake?"

"No," I replied, "I think we need to go to lunch!"

I reminded him that one of his remaining goals was to use up some gift certificates he had to Texas Roadhouse before he "vanished," as he would call it. I don't know how to describe in words what happened that day. Cancer once again blessed Sandi and me for being part of God's plan by witnessing a miracle. I recommend it. They are incredible to see!

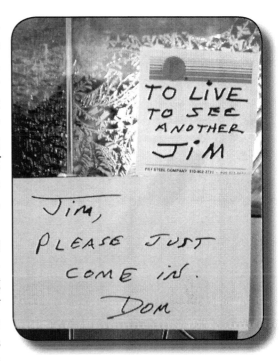

I challenged my dying warrior to fight that day. He had never quit anything before in his life. On my watch, he would not quit on me. I knew that defeat was the cancer talking. I also knew Who my friend had in his heart. He had the same power that raised the one he prays to from his own deathbed. We started talking about positive things like faith and family, fight and fun and the bond that Dom and I shared. How we'd come this far against all odds and statistics. Dom now sat up, his strength building.

"Jim, you're right," he said. "Why let it get me down? We are all appointed to die someday, but why should I die today?"

I was hearing the heart of a warrior kick in for another round.

"I get so down with this cancer, it wears on you," he said. "After a while it's got me and I'm not fighting anymore. What am I doing? Hey Jim, I'm your little Italian Stallion, right? No way cancer, I am living today so I can see another sunrise tomorrow."

"Dom, are you hungry? We need to get you some lunch. Are those gift certificates still good?"

Patt pulled me aside.

"Are you sure we should do this?"

"We have to do it, Patt. It has nothing to do with him eating, but everything to do with him going. Faith is an "F" word that requires action. Two hours ago, he couldn't talk or walk and now he's taking us to lunch. He is a fighter, we are his corner, it's the last round and we win this round."

The four of us settled into our booth at Texas Roadhouse. Tears poured down my checks. I wished I had a magic wand to wave and heal us all. I was humbled that God would allow a mess like me to be here at all. I marveled at how faith and a fighter's heart can accomplish the impossible.

Everyone in that restaurant had no clue a miracle was happening right before their eyes. We are all so busy with life that we often miss its truest meaning. *For their eyes and ears are open, but cannot see or hear.* I prayed for those around our table before my Dom reached across the table to take our hands into his.

Dom, as only he could pray, asked his Lord to bless our "last supper." His words of faith, hope and joy were so filled with passion that it was dripping off of them. The prayer of a righteous man is powerful and effective. The whole restaurant became silent as I listened to his heartfelt words of love and commitment as he thanked God, yes, thanked God, for allowing cancer to use us both for good. Dom prayed that he had been blessed his whole life and would be forever grateful that God saved a sinner.

Readers, I have been around church people a long time, and by far the most powerful words ever spoken for my ears was this prayer from a dying cancer warrior who refused to give in or give up.

Two days after our "last supper," Patt asked if I could come quickly to see Dom. She warned me he was on the portable toilet set up in their living room next to the hospice bed. That's the reality of things.

"Could you wait a bit?" she asked. "I'd like to clean him up and spray some freshener."

"Thank you, Patt. I am a warrior, and a warrior does what a warrior does."

I waited a few minutes.

"Please, go ask Dom if he is okay with me coming in now."

She reopened the door. Dom laid eyes on me and I knew from my years of staring cancer in the face that time was running short.

Dom was a fellow warrior, a fighter, a brother and a mentor. He made a point of getting dressed every day, even when he was so weak he couldn't pull his socks up. Only at the very end did I ever see Dom in bed, and that, my friends, is the heart of a warrior.

He leaned on me for balance while I tore strips of the toilet paper, rearranged his gown and kept his oxygen tubes from tangling and hooking on something as Patt and I helped him back onto the bed. I was lost for words for what was in my mind and heart. For the last time, I was holding his hand, hugging him and kissing his forehead. All he could think of was his concern for Patt. He did not want to die and leave her a mess to clean up. Patt wanted to care for him till the end; she is the warrior of caregivers. Sandi and Patt should be caregivers of the year!

My fellow warrior was going home to be completely healed and renewed. My heart broken and eyes blurry with tears, we spoke slowly and quietly. I could tell he was trying to ask me a question, and I bent close to his mouth to hear.

Slowly and with much effort, Dom said, "I love you Jim, would you have wiped my butt if I asked?" Classic Dom right until the end. He knew I would have done anything for him, and with a twinkle still in his eye, he acknowledged our deep friendship.

As I left the house, I knew I would not visit him again. He needed his family and my time was over. Crying so hard while driving back home, broken again by cancer, I was lost for words and my heart hurt too much to speak.

Dom had a new nickname, "Heart of a Warrior." When the phone rang early the next morning with the news, I began crying again, but this time it was tears of joy, because the Italian Stallion was finally whole again. I knew he was up there hustling someone new to fight him.

I thanked God that I witnessed another sunrise that morning, but this one was especially bright because I know God was delighted to have his warrior home.

For many months after Dom's death, Patt and I struggled to revisit. I find it very difficult with some spouses to carry on our relationship. Just looking at each other, all we do is cry. We did regroup, and bless her heart, we still enjoy our time together, sad, yes, but delighted in knowing our fellow warrior died fighting in faith.

Patt shared with me that on Dom's last night she slept by her husband's side. Moving the toilet out of the way, she maneuvered the living room couch close by. She adjusted the hospice bed to a lower level to be as close as possible, and spent a long night listening to his labored, rattled breathing.

She told me that around four in the morning he softly called for her assistance. He wanted help to be moved to the nearby toilet. Supremely exhausted, he struggled to empty himself. He whispered his last words to thank his loyal teammate for her unconditional love. Dom's final love and concern for his wife was granted that morning. She had no mess to clean up and Dom died sitting upright in her loving arms.

Our brave warrior left us in 2014. I have struggled mightily to cope without his powerful prayers and his sense of humor. Yet in his honor, I move forward to help others like he helped me. Dom showed us all that absolutely, without doubt or question, to survive or to die with honor, you must have the heart of a warrior.

Here, I share Dom's final email to me and fellow warriors, which included a link to a video of Dolly Parton singing "Swing Low, Sweet Chariot." It also had a picture of the memorial marker he had already prepared, a cross bearing this verse from Psalm 49:15: "For God will redeem my soul from the power of the grave; for He shall receive me."

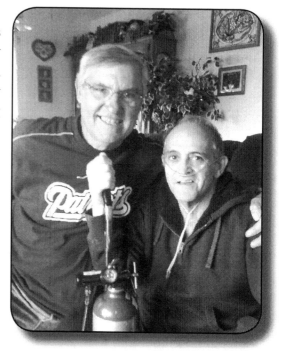

It was a good fight, but how do you fight your own body? Just so you know, I received a call from my doctor today which confirmed my worst suspicions. There is nothing more they can do for me. I have to admit, they gave it their best shot and all the extra stuff I did... well, nothing worked, not theirs and not mine. They are taking all of my medications away because they aren't working and sending me to end of life hospice care. Hospice will only take those not on any medication or doctor's care and are given up by their doctors. I have only weeks left to live at this point.

To those of you who have prayed for me, Thank You So Much. Your prayers gave me hope till the very end. I have asked that nothing be done, no fanfare, no celebration of my life, just the family taking my cremated ashes to be placed on the hill above my home, where I have prepared my grave site eight years ago.

I am not upset, I have lived a long and happy life. I just wish I could stay longer to be with my wife and family, but God wants me with Him. This will be the most glorious trip of my life, entering onto eternity with the Lord Jesus Christ my savior, whom I have known since I was eleven years of age. He has never left my side. Do not be sad for me, but be happy. Thank you all for being my friends on this earth. I hope to see you up there. Whatever you do, please don't miss Heaven.

-Dom

THAT WARRIOR'S HEART

Here's what Dom would want us all to know: When life is going well we can fall into the trap of believing that good times will never end. But when sudden tragedy or death confronts us, we can be shaken to our very core. But facing the fact of life's brevity can help us do a better job of living the time that is allotted to us.

Life is on loan from God. Therefore, we do well to understand as much as we can of its length and breadth, its strength and weakness and its place in human history. By fighting with the heart of a warrior when we die, or survive, either way we honor our families.

In every new visit to a cancer patient, the first thing I listen for is that "heart of a warrior" language. I know it by how it fires up my own heart.

If you already consider yourself dead, now that the big "C" is on your forehead, do you realize everyone can hear that? Will your unfaithful negative words inspire or encourage your loved ones on your team? Are they helping you?

Sadly, more than you would think, I hear defeat, doubt and discouragement in those hospital rooms. I have attended too many funerals for people who talked like this on our first visit. I pray I can help them realize that their words and their inner attitude help everyone involved. One of the greatest compliments I got from my family is when they shared, "never once did we hear Jim complain or be negative."

May I suggest from my experience that the "Big C" qualifies you for a warrior's heart? Something small yet significant sets apart two mindsets; that is, the heart of the weak from the heart of a warrior. One quits at tragedy and the other just begins. The weak-hearted see the day of diagnosis as the day of disaster, but the warrior heart sees every day as a day of triumph. It's your decision.

The weak at heart take their cancer upon themselves to defeat and overcome, only to be overcome. It becomes their identity and over time, because of cancer's relentlessness, they give in and give up, stifling any chance of faith and hope and allowing only total fear and darkness.

The warrior heart, by contrast, uses tragedy to move forward into the unseen and understands even if you don't. By seeing things that are not as though they were, they keep open the hope by faith that their fight will be won, and light will shine not only on them but their loved ones also, even in death.

Little Dom won every fight, not with a big right hook, but with an unseen, but not unheard, heart of a warrior. We must fight for life. Is it precious to you?

Cancer could care less how good you look on the outside. It wants to kill you from the inside out. Don't stay in your corner at the bell. Get off your butt and kick its ass with the heart of a warrior!

I did, Dom did, young David did, and you can too! YOU HAVE THE TOOLS AND THE HEART NOW!

Warrior Words – Chuck

Hi Jim, hope this note finds you well and happy. Just thought I would let you know what happened with my last visit to the doctor. He said they looked at all my old scans and compared them with the new one. They found no bad guys in the attic. Doc said he considered me one in a million because I was doing well and I was still alive. He asked me how I did it and I immediately told him about you and what you did for me.

The last doctor I saw said I was amazing and he couldn't believe what good shape I was in for having what I did. He said he had never seen anyone in all his history of Glio patients look as good as I do at this point. So thanks so much for all your positive waves. You are the miracle worker. I felt good about the news the doctor gave me but I felt even better on Saturday. I went trap shooting with my new fancy Beretta. I was shooting 11s and 12s when I first got it. I was a double A shooter before the cancer showed up. Saturday, I shot a 22 and a 23 so that made me feel like I was moving back toward normal. Thanks to my mentor, I got my port on the left side so I can shoot. You're so smart! I go back for a checkup scan around Christmas. My daughter is about three or four weeks from having what I hope will be my first granddaughter or my second grandson – we will see. Hope you're having a great summer. Be well!

-Chuck

CHAPTER 10

The Smell of Smoke and Fresh Soil

HOPE is such a marvelous thing.

It bends, it twists, it sometime hides, but rarely does it break. It gives us reason to continue and courage to move ahead, when we tell ourselves we'd rather give in.

HOPE puts a smile on our face when the heart cannot manage. It puts our feet on the path when our eyes cannot see it.

HOPE moves us to act when our souls are confused.

HOPE is something to be cherished and nurtured, and something that will refresh us in return. It can be found in each of us, and it can bring light into the darkest of places.

NEVER LOSE HOPE!

THE REAL WALKING DEAD

I know many warriors who are not cancer patients. There's a middle-aged man with a heart transplant, a couple whose 20-year-old son was killed by a drunk driver, a young lady addicted to drugs, a woman suffering from mental and physical punishment, a dear warrior raped by her father and uncle by age eighteen.

Who's really the sickest? Those battling illness, or the rest of society?

Over the past few years, I've met many other battle-worn souls. I've been honored to meet these valiant warriors, and together we vow to finish the fight. We all agree, no matter the tragedy, you cannot quit.

One thing I hear from all honest warriors is how their tragedy, though difficult, renewed their outlook on life and death, sunrise, sunsets, and heaven and hell. What else is there?

Cancer turns our eyes back to the Creator; where before cancer, we often exchanged the truth for a lie and worshiped and served other things. We thought we had eyes to see but now realize it's all smoke and mirrors. We thought we had ears to hear, but realize now that without true love, this world's chatter, gossip and "Entertainment Tonight" are worthless and nothing more than a clanging cymbal.

I love the fact that cancer cut out the crap of this world and simplified my life down to each sunrise and sunset. My family team has a new view of this world, too, a new "attitude of gratitude." We have all been humbled, which always makes you better.

Some warriors don't want help if they are not desperate. I have found we must stay desperate to be healed. Why? Because it keeps us desperate for the grace in which we now stand. Desperate is rewarding, for it keeps our eyes focused on the invisible and unseen.

I have learned, and continue to learn, new lessons on pride as I move forward with my battle. *(Daniel 4:37)* Every hard lesson humbled me lower and even lower until, finally, I was low enough to be lifted up in humility. Listen to me please: Great successes often harden sinners' hearts and make them more daring. Pride only destroys, it cannot heal or make new. I have been to a lot of funerals to prove it. Pride blinds our eyes and steals our dreams. May the light of the rainbow in the dark set us free instead.

SMELL THAT SMOKE?

Many warriors have touched my life and made me a better everything. I owe them for being patient with me, yet getting in my face when I need it most. They keep me on task and reward me with their wonderfully grateful, focused attitude. Again, I could write a whole book on my living warriors. For this chapter, I choose just three. Thank you for encouraging me. I love you all.

In the spring of 2011, I met a newly diagnosed brain cancer warrior named Chuck. His boss, Todd, invited me to have lunch with them both.

I met Todd when he and and his wife attended the 2009 Festival of Trees Gala held every year at an elegant location, The Coeur d'Alene Resort next to the lake. I was the spokesperson for a new cancer facility to open in Post Falls.

"You really touched my heart," Todd had told me after my presentation. "I thought of my mom when first I heard you speaking. When Chuck disclosed he now has cancer, you immediately came to mind."

Todd had bought Chuck my first book to read, so he had some clue how messed up I really am. After hellos and chit-chat, Todd broke the ice by asking Chuck how he felt about now being a cancer warrior. Chuck responded immediately:

"My doc says I'm a walking dead man. She says go home and get your personal stuff in order."

What? I was frustrated beyond belief. *Why do doctors make these kind of statements?* The first thing about cancer that Chuck heard was, YOU'RE DEAD!

He invited me to share some of my story, asked how I was doing, what treatments I was on and what hope I had for my future.

"Chuck, I have another sunrise to see, tomorrow! Cancer might kill me someday, but I guarantee you it's not today. I have been saying that for seven years now. I hope you can believe that way, too."

I went on trying to reassure him that I was given no odds to live either, and filled his ears with the impossible goals my team achieved. Chuck kept telling Todd and I which parts of the book "Really got me thinking." He was still working at this time. It was evident that he loved his work and his boss.

"Chuck, what does your future hold?" I asked the walking dead man. He paused.

"'I'm not planning anything, why should I? My wife died of cancer so I know what that looks like. Now it's my turn. I guess we all have to die sometime, but my time came a lot sooner than I would like."

"Chuck, if you had to pick only one thing, what's your first love?"

"Jim, I really like to mess around in my garden."

"Well," I asked, "Do you a have a garden planted for this season?"

"I was planning one, but now, why? I'm a dead man. I can't do anything and I have no time. I won't be here to eat anything, and it'll all go to waste."

"Chuck, my fellow warrior," I said with vigor. "I want you to go home and start a garden, now. If you need help, call me. I don't care if it's one seed or ten acres of seeds. Just PLANT A GARDEN!"

A week later I called Chuck, partly to see how he was doing and invite him to coffee. But, way more importantly, I was impatient to know the truth: had he planted a garden? Had he done anything beside stay in his chair thinking about being DEAD?

"Coffee sounds great," Chuck said. "I can't believe you called so soon. That's really nice of you, Jim."

"Chuck, I want to be on your team," I said. "I have been where you are and want to help you maneuver around cancer's traps."

"I finished your book," he said. "Man, you're strong! I appreciate you checking on me. I'm doing okay, I have a ton of tests coming up and will start radiation soon. So far I'm handling my cancer and just trying to sort everything out. Thank you for meeting with my boss and me; do I have a great boss or what?"

Nothing about the garden. I was discouraged that he'd forgotten our plan after all.

"Well Chuck, thanks for your time. See you Friday?"

"You bet Jim"

"Okay, Chuck take ca…..."

"Oh, by the way, Jim. I took your advice, went to Ace Hardware, bought some tomato plants and planted some seeds. The work made me feel good. You are like my drill sergeant, and you keep me in line. You're a good guy to have on my team."

On my end of the phone call, I pumped my fist in the air. YES!

I'm not a doctor, and I only know what I have lived and experienced. I was vastly concerned for Chuck because he had "dead" on his brain. I wanted him to engage, to quit talking and thinking death, and to think about fresh new life, instead. Right or wrong, this is how I see it. I'm a survivor! Pick your plan!

Chuck had been pushed deep into soil that smelled of death. There, he had to decide whether to die in the dark or grow up toward the light. Just remember, my friend, the deeper down you go, the better the root system you develop for whatever life may throw at you next.

Don't let cancer plant you. Instead, plant your garden!

Whether you are a cancer warrior or not, the best way to predict your future is to help create it. What's your first love? ENGAGE AND DO IT!

Chuck is a self-proclaimed simple guy. I'd call him a genius. He developed products at his plant that no one else has, but many people want. He took me on tours of the facility and I was amazed at what he knew. He'd worked there 35 years and was getting close to retiring. Right.

"Jim, I'm cutting way back on hours," he would say, which to him meant 50 a week. He's a crazy warrior and that's why we like each other.

Chuck spent months training a new employee to take his place, saying "I want everything done right when I'm gone from here."

Chuck and I enjoy encouraging and holding each other up. He's one of five or so warrior battle buddies I call "cancer survivors and survivors of cancer." They are double survivors, because they have fought their own cancer, and that of a loved one, too. To top everything off, his daughter is my grandson's teacher. How great is that?

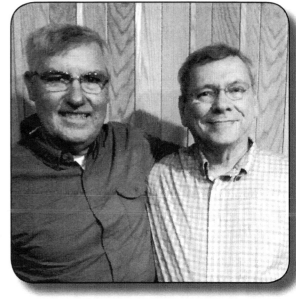

Sandi and I were invited to Chuck's retirement party. What an honor to witness such an event. Proof again that we should NEVER LOSE HOPE! It was a surprise dinner party at a wonderful country club, and they put on a spread.

I had a chance to meet his work mates, who all agreed that Chuck is the real deal. I was humbled how many of his fellow employees knew who I was. "You're Chuck's drill sergeant," they said. It brought joy to my heart to watch Chuck shine in his moment, with the words "walking dead man" ringing in my mind.

Chuck received a beautiful Italian side-by-side shotgun for his other favorite hobby, shooting trap. The party, full of fun, tears and excitement, was a truly fitting end to a brilliant career. Now Chuck's new career is full-time cancer warrior. *Evil cancer, you put your saddle on the wrong horse again. You're bucked off!*

I will always believe my life was extended for just one person. And because I never know who, when or where this "one" is present, I thank God for every warrior with whom I can share my story.

One fall evening, after one of our community cancer group meetings, where I'd handpicked him for my leadership team, Chuck stopped me in mid-step on the way back to the car.

"Jim, smell the smoke from that fireplace? You know, I'm so grateful for the wonderful smell of smoke from a hardwood fire, and when I'm working my garden in the spring, ah, the smell of newly-turned soil, how fresh everything is again."

He has had some problems with his cancer, a reoccurrence which required Gamma knife, and has had symptoms of fatigue, along with "chemo brain." But my friend has the heart of a warrior. Today, that walking dead man feeds plenty of people from his thriving garden. He's so crazy with this garden stuff, especially now that he's retired, that he recently removed the kids' old standup pool, trampoline and anything else from his backyard to give him more ground to plant.

Lesson learned: Watch what you say to warriors! Don't ever tell them they are through. While Chuck now plants many large seeds in his garden, he once upon a time had faith the size of one very small mustard seed… And that was enough.

THE TRUEST HUNT OF ALL

I am a hunter who was brought up in the traditions of a hunting family. I remember some great times hunting with my dad. My son, Jeff, is a diehard bird hunter. He could care less about big game, but he is addicted to waterfowl. Now my grandson Byron is old enough to share that hunting tradition, and it makes me very happy.

Hunting got me through some bleak times, when Jeff and I shared some precious days together in a boat blind while I was in the midst of my cancer fight, unsure of the future, frail and bald.

I really enjoy hunting for mule deer. Near my home in Idaho, we are blessed to have a decent population. And since I'm only two hours south of the Canadian border, I often travel up there to hunt.

During the hunting season of November, 2012, I had a guided mule deer hunt planned in southern Idaho. This is a very difficult tag to draw. I was really excited for the chance of taking a big mule deer and completing another goal on my "things to accomplish in my future" list.

After the eight-hour drive, I arrived at the outfitter's lodge. I begin preparing all hunting equipment for the next day's ride into remote mountains. That fall, the weather was extremely hot, with no snow or even a break in the weather for weeks. Aaron, my guide, was as well aware as I was that this makes for tough hunting.

On the way to hunting camp, we didn't see a single deer. And as the hot, windless days drew on, the sightings did not improve much.

Aaron suggested that I return home, wait until it snowed, then head back to complete my hunt. My guide knew the size of buck I was hunting for and didn't want to waste our time looking for him in less-than-ideal conditions. We broke camp and returned to the lodge.

Just before I'd left for the trip, I had received my initial shipment of my first book, *To See Another Sunrise*. I'd wondered how many to pack, and for some reason I'd brought two. I'd handed Aaron one earlier on my arrival, and now he wouldn't quit talking about it.

"But how do you visit everybody?" he asked me.

"Well, it's time consuming for sure, but one by one I do my best to visit them all."

After we sat and talked for a while longer, I sensed he needed to ask me a question but was hesitant to do so.

"Jim, could I ask a favor of you?"

"Sure, what's up?"

"A good friend of mine just received word his wife has cancer. Could you…"

"Yes, let's go!"

Now I knew why I'd brought two books. Grabbing the other book, we headed to Kelly and Kim's house, a very nice place out in the middle of nowhere. I loved it.

Aaron introduced me to his friends and our conversation began. Kim was very anxious and concerned about her cancer, but after discussing some heavy stuff, she seemed more at ease. I signed her copy of the book and presented it to her.

"Kim, I'm leaving for home but I will soon return to finish my hunt," I said. "Please read this book and see if it can help you. Also, I'll bring you another present."

"Come back and we'll all have dinner together," she replied.

I love driving time. As I got behind the wheel and made the long, but scenic drive home, I kept Kim in my thoughts and prayers.

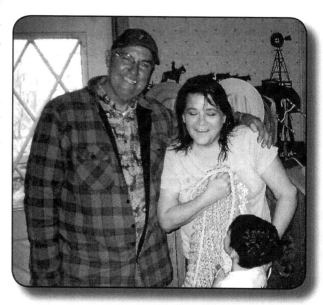

As promised, I returned three weeks later. When I saw Kim, she ran up and gave me an incredible bear hug.

"What's that for?" I asked.

"Jim, I read your book, and I will be a survivor!"

Another fist pump. YES!

"Kim, here is your present that I promised."

I pulled a beautiful hand-stitched lap blanket from the box, and she melted. With both of us crying now, it was my turn to give her a bear hug.

"This is for you, warrior. Some dear sweet women in my church weave these for my warriors. They want you to know they care and they handmade this just for you. Kim, I am so impressed by your attitude and your focus on planning your future. You have a dedicated team with you, now take the field, girl!"

Two days later, I was sitting on an outcropping of rock in the Idaho backcountry, watching the storm clouds finally blowing in. This was the weather we'd been counting on to bring snow and cold and get the deer moving.

I pondered again how blessed I felt to have been spared and now to help others. The Bible makes it clear that being selfish doesn't help you to become rich. Freely you have received, freely give. God has showered his blessings on me, and that means I should give generously to others my time, love and possessions. I was amused and amazed by how the focus of this hunt had been detoured to God's will.

From my elevated perch, with binoculars in hand, I saw nothing that looked like a buck. The clouds rolled around me in shades of purple, grey and blue. I thought of the incredible storms I'd seen over the years, both the ones in nature and the ones in life.

I dug through my pack for the camera, intent on capturing this surreal setting. I was seated close to the edge of a canyon looking into treetops right in front of me. *What kind of a climb it would be if you found yourself in a hole like that? What if you got injured and needed help? No one could hear your screams. You'd be on your own to survive, or die.* That hole was my cancer fight.

As I sat and pondered, it was like someone threw a switch. Nearly instantly, the sun broke out and an incredible double rainbow appeared. *WOW! SHOWTIME!*

As I sat alone on that mountain, in awe of these powerful colors overhead, I realized once again how small I was in the real scope of this universe. I'd waited six years to draw this tag and hunt this area. But in my heart I knew there was way more going on here than mule deer hunting. I knew that rainbows stand for promises kept, and this one re-assured me that His promises are real and last for eternity.

My goal for the trophy buck is still in my focus and future. Your friend Jim Morrison accomplishes goals and this one is no different. But until the next hunting oppor-tunity, I am content to cherish my trophy from this hunt. I have met a fellow warrior with a tough team, and that's a moment in time with real meaning forever. Perhaps now this hunt can inspire you to pursue your goals and plant your garden.

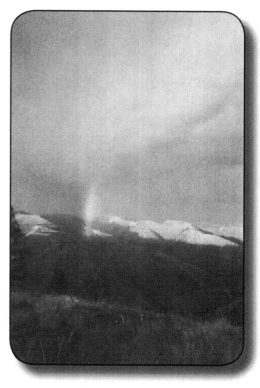

Some diehard hunters would think I wasted a lot of time and money for nothing. Why would I spend that hunt talking, delivering gifts and eating instead of pursuing my quarry?

This I know: as a cancer survivor, my views and goals are much different than they used to be. Those trophy antlers with a big score hanging in the game room will never match the trophy I received. I am reminded of that fact every time Kim calls to say, "Thank you Jim, I am NED four years now. I want you to know I have seen many sunrises. I can't wait to share those sunrises, and a rainbow, with you in heaven."

MISSILE LOCK

It was a beautiful summer day and I was preparing for a meet-and-greet book signing at our local Bible bookstore. I'd set up the table and hung signs, and now I sat marveling, as I always do post-cancer, at the little details of the moment: the warm coffee mug in my hand and the big blue sky outside the pane glass window.

I prayed the same prayer I do at each event: *Please Lord, let one, just one person, be here today that especially needs your hope and encouragement. Amen!*

My eyes met a missile lock with the eyes of a man pacing outside the store. I felt with a force he was the answer to my prayers. Finally, he whipped the door open and headed straight to me. I stood to greet him, and saw tears in his eyes. *Yes, he's the one. Thank you, Lord!*

I normally don't do this, but this time, I walked around the table to him and gave him a tight hug, with his biker jacket and all. Standing close, I could feel the hurt. This man was broken, and I didn't know why, but I knew this was show time.

"I'm Jim Morrison, author of *To See Another Sunrise*," I said. "What's your name?"

"Thank you," he said.

"I'm sorry?"

"Thank you," he repeated.

"Man, are you all right? Let me get you some coffee."

"Jim, thank you, again."

I knew from experience, although this day's book sales might be nil, I now had more important unseen matters at hand.

"Sir, if it's okay by you, let's go sit down in the coffee bar area and talk," I said. "I want to know why you are here."

I found the quietest corner and pulled two chairs together.

"Jim, my name is John, and I'm here to buy one of your books for my daughter."

"Hi, John. Is your daughter struggling with cancer?"

"I wish," he said.

What? I wondered how that could possibly be, and where this was going.

"She is addicted to drugs," he said with a heavy heart.

"Why did you come here today, John?"

"My baby girl is in jail," he said.

He told me how he had pressed charges against his own daughter for stealing items from his house and business. He said she had left him no choice. "I just wanted her off drugs," he said.

"But three nights ago, in jail, she was reading a local Christian paper and came across your ad for today's book signing. She wrote a letter begging me. I was freaked out so I went to visit her, and crying and desperate, she told me she needed to have your book. She said, 'If this Jim guy can overcome death, I can beat my addiction.'"

Wow, everything else in the world paled by comparison. Those words were priceless.

"Jim, I drove 10 hours straight to get here. Can I buy a book?"

"John, of course. What can I do to help?"

"The book is all I came for," he said. "I will do anything to get my baby back. I miss her so bad not being here with me."

"John, please don't move, I'll be right back."

Grabbing a book off the table, I had to excuse myself from the six or so others waiting in line to meet me and get their own book.

"What is your daughter's name?"

I opened the book and wrote these words: *To Chelsea, may my story help you write yours someday. Mail me and I will help you if I can. Your fellow warrior, Jim.*

John had the heart of a warrior. Being a parent myself and an adult child of an alcoholic, I knew it's easy to quit on our loved ones. We struggle with doubt when things don't go the way we planned. He could have left her in jail, since she'd brought it on herself, *(Daniel 5:23)* but his daughter's plea for help in her desperate place spurred this father-warrior into action.

I have stayed in touch with John and Chelsea over the years now. When the idea of this new book began, this story was a must-print.

I could tell you the rest of this amazing story myself, but instead, I asked John and Chelsea to finish it. Please read their Warrior Words that follow, and see how the rainbow can guide through any darkness and difficulty. I love them both for their effort to engage and allowing me to be part of their real-life issues. Again, without my cancer, we would have never shared this precious moment, and together found that starting at tragedy leads to triumph. *Thank you, cancer!*

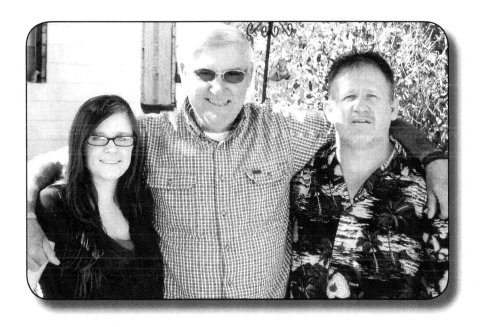

Warrior Words – Chelsea

Eighteen years old, and my life was going great. I was a very young mother to a beautiful little boy. I was working full time, had a house, car and was raising my sweet Davian on my own. One day that all changed.

I started hanging out with my old friends and started doing drugs. Within weeks I quit my job, spent all my saved money and gave up my life and my son. I started using heroin. I was too scared to be around my son. I loved him with every piece of my heart, but drugs are powerful. About a week later I was introduced to meth. I'd never seen it before in my life until the day it was offered to me by my best friend. I tried it and that was it. It's true, that saying, "Meth, Not even once." I was hooked. At that point I asked my mom if she would take care of my son and explained why. She was heartbroken.

From there I quickly went downhill. I met lots of new (bad) people, stopped sleeping and eating. I lost forty pounds in a short two months, weighing just under 100 pounds. My so-called friends found out my dad was out of town and robbed his house and shop. I found out from my mom that they thought I had something to do with it. I had no idea, but who would believe an active meth addict?

I left for Boise with my dad so I could go to rehab. I needed to get sober! Boise was a terrible idea, though. I met up with some not-so-good cousins and fell further into my addiction. I didn't make it to rehab.

After a while the drugs weren't getting me high anymore, so I started using intravenously. It was like nothing I've ever felt before. It was scary, but I could not go back after that experience. While I was in Boise, my friends were at my place in Coeur d'Alene destroying my car and my home, and I had no idea. Finally, I made it back home by bus but had no car and an eviction notice. I got in countless arguments with my parents and was so bad into meth that I literally felt no emotions. I was heartless.

I wanted so badly to be sober and to get my life back. Little did I know it was not going to be so easy. After being evicted I had nowhere to go, I was homeless for a month. I hardly ever slept, but when I did it was either at some random drug house or outside. My parents would not let me stay at either of their houses, but who could blame them? That's when I signed myself into rehab at Port of Hope. But when my mom took me there I just couldn't go. I was scared to get sober now and I was scared to lose all my new "friends."

When I finally decided to go in, my good sober friends convinced me it was the right thing to do. It lasted one week, then I checked myself out. (This is a 30-day inpatient treatment program). I stayed with a friend that night and woke up to his uncle staring at me and trying to pull my top off. I was so scared.

Staying sober didn't last long. This time I had used more meth than I ever did at once and it ruined me forever. I blacked out. I went to my dad's to shower and started seeing and feeling bugs all over me. I dug at myself and cried and didn't understand what was going on. They felt and looked so real. My dad yelled at me to the point he lost his voice. I didn't hear a word that came out of his mouth, though. He had me dropped off at rehab once again. They said my heart rate was so fast I could have had a heart attack if it didn't go down. Then later I could have had a stroke if it wouldn't go back up. Talk about scary!

I left rehab again less than a week later and still felt the bugs. At this point my dad decided to press charges on me for the theft at his house and shop. I got arrested a couple days later. In jail I went to a Bible study and that's when I accepted Jesus Christ back into my life after not believing for about five years or so.

I felt like a new person, praying and reading my Bible all day, every day! I got ahold of a local Christian newspaper, "The Good News." That's where I saw Jim Morrison's story about being a stage 4 cancer survivor and that he had written a book. He was going to be at Sower Bible Book store for book signings. I wouldn't be out in time and I needed that book! So I wrote my dad a letter and asked him to please go get it for me, that it would mean so much to me, so he did. He got me Jim's book and got it signed! I was so happy; God was good!

God is the only reason I got through that month of jail. I had never in my life been in trouble before. After I got out of jail, I was good. I stayed with my mom and my son, who had just turned two, and life was great!

But my goodness, I had no friends, none! I stayed sober for about one more month, then started using again. I never went back to using intravenously though. I didn't get anything done the courts asked me to, and I was on the run for a couple months. I continued using drugs until March 18, 2013. That is the day my life forever changed.

I was arrested again, and this time I was sentenced to a rider, which is basically drug treatment jail for three, six or nine months. Since it was my first offense I got the three-month rider. I completed several classes and learned so much. I went to church every Sunday and read my Bible every day. I set many goals for myself, and I've now achieved several of them. I got to finally meet Jim Morrison, and even now run into him at my home church, Heart of the City.

He is a great guy and was a huge part in me re-believing in Jesus by reading his story in the newspaper that day. As of two days ago, March 18th 2016, I can proudly say I am three years sober and I could not be happier. I have two handsome sons and another son on the way. I know my family is proud of me and how far I've come. I never thought I would make it out of my addiction alive, and I owe it all to God for giving me another chance at this life. My advice for anyone struggling with addiction: do not give up on yourself, and never be afraid to ask for help. Everyone matters and never forget,

YOU ARE LOVED!

-Chelsea

Warrior Words – John

This all started from a letter I received from my daughter, Chelsea, while she was incarcerated in the Kootenai County jail. Chelsea sent me a letter and asked if I would go and buy this book she had learned about, written by Jim Morrison, called *To See Another Sunrise.*

I met Jim at Sower Bible Bookstore, and I was pretty emotional sharing my story with him about Chelsea and her addiction and jail. Jim for some reason knew how broken I was. He was feeling my pain through my words. I as well was touched by his. He knew we were supposed to meet. I shared with Jim how Chelsea was sitting in jail waiting for sentencing. This all started from bad choices and wrong friends. I had been on a trip when my daughter called and asked, 'Daddy when are you coming back home?' I didn't think much of the question but told her when I'd return.

My home and business are on the same property. One of the first things I do by routine is to check in my shop. I made it one step and knew someone had been in there. With certain things out of place and items missing, my heart sank. The first person to come to mind was Chelsea. I went into my house and found things out of place, and I was certain my daughter had something to do with this.

As a parent I was deeply hurt that one of my own children would steal and allow others to do the same. All I wanted was for her to get addiction help. She agreed but wanted to go to Boise to receive help. Chelsea and I headed to Boise, and she took off. I ended up coming back to Coeur d'Alene alone. Chelsea came back a couple weeks later or so. I told her I just wanted her to get help. She had a two-year-old son by this time. Chelsea agreed to go to Port of Hope in Coeur d'Alene. That lasted about two days. She was not serious about it. She would occasionally come over to my shop high on drugs and I would try to talk sense into her.

The only leverage I had on her was that she had stolen from me, so I decided to press charges on her. I called the police and requested a female officer to come and take my statement. She then met with Chelsea who confessed. Chelsea could not believe I would do that to her. She had left me no choice; I wanted her off drugs.

The day at the court hearing was very emotional for me, knowing my daughter could be serving time in jail. When I took the stand it didn't take two questions and I was in tears, knowing I'd lost my daughter. But I didn't. She was sent to the women's correctional facility in Boise and placed on two year's probation and classes. For me, the end result with tough love not only helped but hopefully taught others to do the same. I care about how my children are as people. And their choices have outcomes. My daughter has since thanked me for saving her. She is now three years sober as of March 18, 2016.

I lost my dad to lung cancer at the age of 47. At the diagnosis, he was given a life sentence of two months. As a family we were not ready for this. One of the things that separates Jim Morrison was when my dad was given his remaining time to live, he sat on the couch waiting to die.

I would ask my dad what he was thinking and how he was feeling, but he would quickly change the topic to car talk. I am a car guy because of him. My dad lived for one more month without hope and determination.

I believe with all my heart if he had met my friend, Jim, he too could have lived another day or week or who knows, with the right mindset, he might even be here today.

Jim, you give people hope and inspiration and an open mind, a reason to live. I want to thank you for our friendship, and the hope you inspired in me the first time we met and each time we see one another. You were given a purpose from God and you are doing awesome! Your friend.

-John

CHAPTER 11

Cancer Discussions

Here are some sayings that hold true in cancer just as much as in life:

"In prosperity our friends know us; in adversity we know our friends."

"It is doubtful whether God can bless a man greatly until he's hurt him deeply."

"When someone allows you to bear his burdens, you have found deep friendship."

"Life is a long lesson in humility."

And here is another bit of advice from yours truly: BE YOUR OWN ADVOCATE!

Please don't screw around with your health. Cancer feeds on the attitude of denial and delay. I ask so many people to go see their doctor, and almost always they reply, "It scares me to visit a doctor; what if it's cancer? I would rather not find out."

I respond, "THANK GOD, IF IT'S CANCER, YOU FOUND IT EARLY."

You know your body better than anyone. If you think something is not right, get checked. Chances are very good it has nothing to do with cancer. Don't start at stage 4 like I did. Though I had no idea of my lung cancer before it was almost too late, I wish now I would have checked my three-month nagging cough.

Don't listen to the TV or what you hear from others. If it is cancer, the longer you procrastinate, the better odds you're giving your evil enemy to kill you. If you have a broken fingernail, I don't give a damn if you ever get it checked – it probably won't kill.

Listen to a cancer patient! Do not mess with this killer! I know a young man who was diagnosed with testicular cancer, yet because of a very early detection and a very simple day surgery, he never experienced chemo, radiation or side effects. Today he is a professional Ironman competitor. I know another gentleman who screwed around with seeing his doctor, and was finally diagnosed with the same cancer, but with metastases. Now, after everything he has gone through he can barely walk. Why? He delayed and denied too long. Beware and stay alert. Early detection is by far your best chance at being a survivor instead of a statistic. And again, if you have lungs, smoker or not, you can get cancer!

MENTORING IS A WIN-WIN

I am so grateful for my mentor, Don. My hunting partner and fellow warrior took me under his wings and helped me establish a positive mindset in a very negative situation. I do my best to follow his example by contacting and offering help to new warriors within the first six weeks after their sentence of cancer.

He had received his one year earlier, and was really struggling when he took mine upon himself. Don and I both were at our wit's end, wondering how to live long enough to attend our daughters' weddings. Future goals are what Don taught me, along with reiterating: "tough times never last, but tough warriors do."

Don and I made up our minds to set impossible goals and never allowed the attitude of giving in or up. Everyone we knew was pulling for us, when they knew in reality we had little chance to accomplish these goals. Don once told me: "Don't listen Jim. You are a survivor. Think like one and push forward like one."

Losing my mentor was so difficult that, at the time, I wasn't sure

I could survive on my own. Don was such a great mentor; we dealt with the reality of cancer, but by faith, focused on our goals, not death. There was no whining or poor me. We never allowed drama or BS in our camp. If it was not going to help or encourage us in our battle, we did not want to hear it or see it, and we never went online to find more depressing news.

Don would say what I needed to hear, like it or not. He did not babysit me or enable me. He fought like hell for me, just like I did for him. We did not quit. Instead, cancer's sickness made us push forward into each other, into our families and into our Lord. Cancer made us better men. I made a promise to Don on his last day that I would reach out and help others like he helped me. Thank you, Don. I love and miss you so much.

I've had many great mentors growing up. Who were the people in your life who encouraged you, showed you the ropes and helped you become the person you are today? Think about individuals who offered you encouragement, shared their experiences and knowledge, and sometimes just listened when you needed to talk. Most successful business people and cancer warriors I know tell me they had mentors along the way who guided and encouraged them. Establishing the right relationship is critical to the mentor/mentee relationship.

How do you know if you're cut out to be a good mentor yourself? My business mentor George shared these five key characteristics of an effective mentor, which he learned from motivational author and speaker Harvey Mackay:

COMMITMENT. Are you willing to dedicate the time and effort necessary to a mentoring relationship?

COURAGE. Do you have the courage to take risks, admit mistakes and let others do the same?

CURIOSITY. If you're always asking questions trying to find out how things work and why, you'll be a good mentor.

COMPASSION. Are you patient with others when they make mistakes? Do you try to understand situations from the other person's point of view? As a mentor, your job isn't to pass judgment but to create opportunities for insight and growth in other people.

COMMUNICATION. Can you explain what works for you and why? Telling a warrior what to do in a specific situation doesn't really teach him or her. You'll be more effective if you communicate as explicitly as you can what strategies and techniques have worked best for you.

I've had the privilege of mentoring many fellow warriors, cancer or not. We all need someone to talk to and share our battles. With some, it consisted of a few meetings. With others, the relationship lasted over months or years.

How do you go about finding a good mentor? I suggest local cancer support groups, church groups or online support. I am in many groups online, swapping tips and faith. The infusion room is war zone, and almost everyone in there would love to talk with you. Cancer talks cancer. Don't sign up to share with someone whose toe is broken. Don't limit yourself to one mentor. You may want to have several mentors to help with different aspects of your life. Mentoring presents a tremendous win-win opportunity.

If you don't have a mentor, find one. Why? Because it heals you both. Only when you take your eyes off your situation do you see the pain in someone else's.

It's powerful and it works, trust me! It's easier when two people are pushing the snowball. Both of them must agree, we're moving forward only!

CHEMO BRAIN IS REAL

I don't get away with chemo brain like I use to. My family doesn't cut me much slack anymore. My kids tell me: "Dad, it's been nine years since you had chemo, no way am I buying it, you can't pull that on me anymore." *Can't you feel the love?*

Yet I do have chemo brain, and every honest cancer warrior you meet, if they have undergone a ton of chemo, will have it too. It's a real medical term and CB can and does cause problems. While patients have been telling their oncologists about their cognitive difficulties for years, most doctors were hesitant to acknowledge the condition. Many warriors I meet with often have shared the same story ten times, but with two or more chemo brains talking we always find it new.

I have to write down everything I must remember. My notes drive Sandi crazy because they are everywhere. So many, that some days while getting the oil changed, I spend the whole time sorting and redoing my notes. And when I forget where I put them, I am lost and nervous. Welcome to cancer land.

I do know a few warriors that were not hired back because their employers felt that "chemo fog" might cause problems with an important project or deadline. Christina Meyers, MD, PhD, director of the neuro-psychology section at M.D. Anderson, says cognitive dysfunction related to cancer treatment has become a burgeoning area of investigation. Myers says that cognitive function issues are seen in survivors "across the board." She has seen it in patients with leukemia, lung and testicular cancers. She estimates about 60 percent of patients she has assessed show a cognitive decline.

"Often the patients look really good, but it's a huge effort. The mental cost to function at that level is very taxing."

Meyers says the most common problems she encounters are lapses in short-term memory, difficulty finding intended words and impaired executive function: the brain capability that is necessary for multitasking and focusing. Other frequent complaints include difficulty reading and trouble with math. Some patients experience a more global sense of mental fatigue. Meyers says research has also shown that chemo brain can include impaired balance and motor skills in some patients where fine motor dexterity and speed of accomplishing manual tasks are affected.

"This kind of impairment can be a stumbling block for someone who wants to go back to college or work," Meyers says.

Reclaim your brain. Cognitive therapy is built on the idea that it's not what you have, who you are or what you are doing that makes you happy or unhappy. It's what you think about.

Living in a haze is how most warriors describe their chemo brain. Like anything in cancer land everybody is different and effects will vary. For me, very short-term memory is the worst. I can remember the roof I was repairing an A/C unit on and what day 30 years ago, but after setting my coffee down to answer the doorbell, for the life of me I can't find the damn cup.

I do believe it may have improved a bit, now that I'm more active and writing books, e-mails and back to life. I know some that have no chemo brain, but the neuropathy in their feet is horrible instead. I'll take chemo brain, thank you.

I am convinced chemo brain is very real and disabling. It irritates me when the people without cancer minimize it and say, "Yeah, I have chemo brain" if they forget something. Those remarks downplay the syndrome's reality. I deal with chemo brain, also I'm now 62, and certainly age is a factor. Nevertheless, even with all the collateral damage from my cancer war, including chemo brain, I am grateful I am still able to witness another sunrise and chase another grandbaby. And remember my fellow warriors, we could have Alzheimer's. There are no side effects for those warriors. God bless them.

QUALITY VS. QUANTITY

This is a very tough subject that sooner or later you should discuss.

My mentor, Don, showed me one approach. With all options exhausted, and no new clinical trials in the very near future, he explored his options.

Don wanted to be at his best for his daughter's wedding, so he decided to end the intense chemotherapy treatments and try to recuperate the strength he needed to fully enjoy this wonderful event. He talked it through with his family and chose this path.

Watching Don at that wedding, and the way he carried himself, was a true testament to a warrior's heart. He set an example for me that day that nothing is impossible. A few months later, my mentor passed to heaven.

Quality vs. quantity is not always a pleasant topic, yet it is an important cancer discussion. Many things must be taken into account. Is more chemo pain worth it for a few more months of non-quality life? What is the warrior's age and health, and the spiritual, emotional, mental and physical condition of the caregiver?

For me, it was quality time with my family that I wanted most. Quantity has no meaning when a person is totally disabled by cancer's relentless destruction. Non-quality life is very depressing to loved ones. I always felt I wanted my family to remember me at full speed ahead, not broken down by the side of the road with the hood up while life passed me by.

In this discussion, it's vital to know that physical life is not the end; a new life awaits those who have witnessed the Light of the World while seeing their rainbow in the dark.

Most families I have accompanied through the process have no regrets on the decision they made. At the last it brings peace.

SURVIVOR'S GUILT

I love mentoring cancer warriors, but I have been deeply hurt time and again when my warriors run out of time. I struggle daily with survivor's guilt.

I become a part of these families. They invite me into their lives and send me Christmas and birthday gifts. I meet everyone in the family, and I know the names of their kids and their pets, their favorite football team, what flavor ice cream they eat, and whether they hunt, fish, hike, bowl, snowmobile, paint or read books. These relationships carry on for awhile after the warrior passes. In time, life takes over again, which it should, and finding time to share becomes more difficult. E-mails and calls are a good way to communicate. I do stay in touch, and most of these families impact me and are a blessing. (There are a very few that I'll never visit again as long as God gives me breath).

Sandi and I have argued at length about my work as a cancer mentor. She tells me, "I thank God for you being a survivor, but your family needs your time and so do I."

I spend hundreds of hours with fellow warriors, often bedside in homes, hospitals, living rooms and hospice facilities. Some I have met and not really had time to learn much about them; it can be that quick. Others I have spent years with, and those are the toughest.

I know three women whose husbands' time ran out. I stay in touch with all, but have yet to meet and discuss with them since the funeral. We can't talk on the phone without crying, so how could we ever meet? From past experience when I look into their eyes I see the loved one they lost and I know the opposite is also true. All of these men and I spent years together sharing cancer, good and bad, and laughing and crying like babies. These relationships are real, priceless and powerful.

My relationship with their wives is tough. In particular, talking to Don's wife Val is still extremely difficult for me. Bless their hearts, these women go out of their way to comfort and reassure me, support my work and share how proud they are of me. They are always so grateful for the wonderful time I shared with their loved one. I am looking forward to the day when we can all meet and cry together, but this time with tears of joy.

This past year I performed and attended more funerals than I can handle. I feel the hurt in the survivors, and I realize again what an impact my death would have made on my family.

I can't do it! My survivor's guilt has become an enormous distraction. It wants to defeat the mission. It causes delay in making the call or visiting the newly diagnosed warrior and their family. Since I don't know if they'll survive or not, why take the chance to be hurt again? I start questioning my motives and my faith. *It seems everyone I'm around dies.*

When I visit a dying warrior for the last time, I am absolutely crushed when I leave. My hope and faith struggles to understand. Still, I don't and won't quit.

Why them and not me? Why does stage 1 die when I was stage 4? She was only 33 years old with babies to raise. How in the world will his spouse handle him being gone after 55 years of marriage? Why spare me, Lord?

When I was first diagnosed, I asked, "Why me?"

Now 12 years later, I'm still asking the same question, but it's come full circle.

"Why did I survive, while so many others did not?"

For me, the answer lies in more important questions: "For who, when and where?"

It takes hours, sometime days of quiet time in prayer and retooling to get my head engaged, and go back to the duty I have been set apart to accomplish. Sandi, bless her heart, knows when I'm hurting, and that my goals come at a price.

I've talked to some who think I'm wasting my time with the walking dead. They suggest I should be doing book signings and speaking engagements, trying to make money instead. *Who's really the sickest?*

This I know! I must put my God and family first, for without them I wouldn't be here to do anything. And I say to every cancer dog from hell nipping at my heels, barking "Guilt, Guilt!" while I am moving forward to mentor another – you will not disable me.

At the end of the day, the wonderful side effects of mentoring can heal you like no medicine in a TV commercial can. I struggle with survivor's guilt, but what a blessing.

Guilt means I'm alive to fight another day, and enlist you, too, to accomplish the impossible so we can be guilty together.

CHAPTER 12

Encouraged to Move Forward

My first contact with Dorothy and Charles came by e-mail. She expressed her thoughts on the book and a recent article about my story in our local newspaper. "My husband Charles would love to meet you, as would I, if at all possible," she wrote.

Driving into town for our first meeting, I was excited as always, but hesitant. In years of meeting now with hundreds of people, I have found, like each cancer is different, so too are first meetings.

As words flowed and thoughts shared, I learned that Dorothy was a career nurse and sees things from a different angle, which is great. She reminded me of my daughter, Kym, who is also a nurse. Both women are of slender frame, yet both "little nurses" can be as sweet as Mother Theresa one minute, or rip your heart out and hand it to you the next.

Charles had five academic degrees and worked as a management and educational consultant. His career had taken him all around the world and he and Dorothy had traveled extensively.

I was amazed to learn that Charles was 79 and a FOUR-time cancer warrior. I had met a few three-time warriors, but he was the first to have beat the enemy four times. We discussed the cancers this warrior had defeated, including: melanoma, carcinoma, prostate and breast cancer. WOW! His first experience was in 1987 when Dorothy, 77, Charles' wife of 45 years, noticed this "awful thing on your arm."

Charles is rare in more ways than one. He is the only man, in nine years of mentoring warriors, I have known with breast cancer. He received chemotherapy and underwent a mastectomy to get rid of that. It was obvious he had the heart of a warrior from the first time I met him.

He invited me to our local community Kroc Center to walk with him on their hardwood track.

"My all-time record is 12 laps," he told me. "Jim, do you think you can stay up with me?"

Charles told me he was feeling "super," but his nurse wife said different. "Charles is weak and frail today," she told me. "We'll see how he does."

As we walked laps, I realized how remarkable it was to share my morning with a four-time survivor. One cancer came very close to killing me. I couldn't imagine four. Nearing the finish line for lap five, Charles said, "Jim, I'm getting tired, can we sit?"

"Sure, you bet."

"Ok, Jim we'll rest now," he said as he continued to walk.

Rounding the corner to start six, I asked him about resting, "One more," he said. Finally, after seven laps, he sat down. I grabbed us some water. I was so impressed with how this guy just pushed himself.

"Charles, thank you so much for inviting me to walk with you. You are an inspiration to be around. Can I help you get ready to leave?"

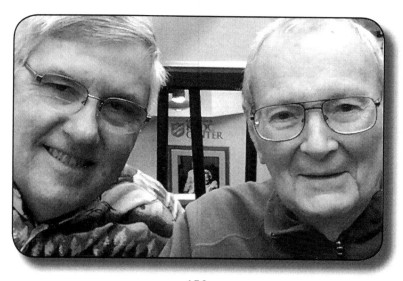

"Yes, Jim, let's do that, I'm feeling very tired and weak."

"That's fine man, you completed seven laps, good job."

Charles stood up, but instead of heading for the exit, he started walking the track again.

"Charles, aren't you done for the day?"

"Yes I am, after one more lap."

WOW! I knew I'd just found my newest mentor. I love it when I meet someone offering my help, and receive encouragement from them instead. That's why I hang out with cancer people.

As of this book, we have walked miles together on this track, and with each encouraging lap I am blessed again to be a part of his personal walk. Charles did run into trouble a year after I met him. He and Dorothy were exercising in the Kroc Center and on the way out he told her he was in terrible pain. Doctors discovered a fracture in his vertebrae.

"When they did the MRI, they found the facture but they also found a tumor on where it fractured." Dorothy told me. "Jim, it truly was a blessing, otherwise we wouldn't have known that he had a growing cancer on his spine."

The final diagnosis; Stage 4 metastatic cancer of the spine. That was cancer number FIVE for my incredible warrior friend.

Instead of Kroc walking, I now visited him in a rehab facility. He struggled some days just to move or get out of bed, yet Charles was still joyful. There was some confusion about meals and medicine one day while I was there. God help the crew now that Dorothy was all fired up! Sitting bedside in his room, Charles and I could both overhear her conversation with the staff six doors away. Caregivers do what caregivers do. Needless to say, this issue was resolved. It's a valuable reminder this is your life, and you should take control of it. If you have a simple sprain, let it go. But we have cancer and it kills! Do not accept a "whatever" approach. Fight for your life! At best we have one shot to get it right. Good facilities, making good decisions at good times, are very important if you are to finish this fight.

Many visits Charles never even saw me. I was happy just to spy on him. I could see the determination on his face as he was engaged in the rehab work room. If he couldn't walk, he could lift arm weights while sitting in his wheelchair. Or bounce a ball against a wall and catch it to help his coordination. He's a warrior and we don't quit. *YES!*

Dorothy would give me very thorough updates on his process. It's much easier to do when you're in the corner of a strong fighter. Beloved Charles was in this facility for many months and, with his kind and gentle personality, really bonded with the staff. When it came time for him to be released, they celebrated with a grand sendoff.

As I write this, tomorrow is Charles' 80th birthday, and I'm selecting a card and balloon I will surprise him with. I'm encouraged that through all the cancer, this warrior beat them all to celebrate another sunrise. I love him and Dorothy for inviting Sandi and me into their battle. We bless each other as only cancer and God can. Our biggest joy now is when we take our impossible granddaughter Jenna to visits with us. Dorothy and Charles just light up when she's there. Charles tells me, "Don't even bother coming over without the baby."

The thought of Charles and I laughing and sharing life should give you massive hope. Here is a stage 4 lung cancer warrior with metastasis to the pericardial lining around his heart hanging out with a FIVE-TIME cancer survivor. Can I get an AMEN?

Charles has lifted my game. I need encouragement to get through the heartache, devastation and funerals I share with warriors and their families. Charles is my rock and my mentor. I look up in

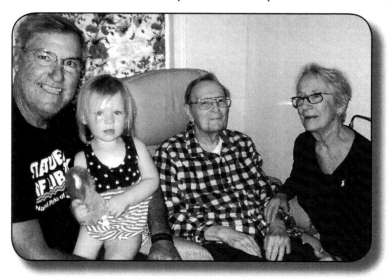

respect and honor to this man. I know how tough this disease is, and yet this 80-years-young warrior fights on like no other I have met. He is truly the Goliath in my cancer world, unbeatable, the heavyweight champ!

Only when God needs his saint will he be gone. I treasure this fellow walking buddy beyond belief. *Walking again? Did you doubt? Oh, ye of little faith!*

This treasure I found because I followed the rainbow up and out of the pit is walking again. Charles and I are lucky now to finish three laps. One lap he's using a cane, the second his walker and the third lap, just his legs. He does it, in spite of odds and statistics.

He does it, and so should you!

Five blows from cancer and Charles is still ticking. Listen to what the heart of a warrior said to me at that very first meeting:

"It never gets easier, Jim, and it's always scary, but I ALWAYS feel I can beat it."

Jenna, Sandi and I look forward to soon delivering another balloon and card that will celebrate 81 years. Through nearly 30 years of knowing cancer, Charles has stayed strong. He speaks softly and grins a lot, and certainly hasn't lost his sense of humor. He teases that he has his wife completely under control and playfully offers to sell me his cat for astronomical amounts of money.

I thank God for Dorothy and Charles, with a very grateful heart, for encouraging me and always supporting the work. That offers hope, and provides an example of strength for the rest of us to KEEP MOVING FORWARD!

STUCK IN NEUTRAL

There's a verse in the Bible that I feel many people don't fully understand: "Consider it pure joy, my brothers, whenever you face trials of many kinds, because you know that the testing of your faith develops perseverance. Perseverance must finish its work so that you may be mature and complete, not lacking anything."

In times of suffering, people sometimes wish they knew the future, or wish they could understand the reason for their anguish. I just realized from writing this chapter that I have discovered another tool, another cherished "F word" in my journey, and that is FUTURE. This one will help me move closer to being mature and complete. FUTURE MEANS FORWARD.

I know from personal experience that talking and thinking about moving forward mentally is very difficult when you can't move physically. I had six months of future. What about Chuck the "walking dead man?" My cancer buds and I have learned this about the future: DON'T LET OTHERS DICTATE YOURS.

Come to our community group and ask Kim, the lady who died on the operating table. She'll set you right!

In cancer, there is no neutral. Forward or reverse is all that remains. Certainly, "Stable" is a good word in cancer world. But I say this also from experience: you don't want to stay there. I found a lot of my future began at stable. I had to be thinking, and working my butt off, to move forward to stable. But getting that stable report was not enough for me. It's cancer; do you think it quits trying to steal your future because you're stable?

From where you are now, looking into your future may make you angry, because you feel you don't have one. Just remember, my friend, that fear or faith dictates your future. It takes a ton of energy to become a survivor, so don't waste any on being negative. Be aware of deception and diversion and stay focused on your future goals. Anything but that could be your downfall.

Fear and faith work like the old snowball effect. Remember as kids how we started rolling a very small snowball? By pushing and positive energy, the ball grew bigger and bigger until it became huge.

I have been overwhelmed in my new future by faith. Fearful yes, through the trials and tribulations and much testing and hardship. But it is possible to profit from them and turn these tragic times into times of learning. Tough times can teach us perseverance.

I can't imagine how overwhelming these trials and hardships must be when engaged with only fear, and without faith as a weapon.

I believe us cancer warriors should help prepare and shape the future for our caregivers and loved ones by our example. Survive or not, future-forward, requires us to be always on the move. I would never allow my team to know that their dad/husband/friend just quit at tragedy. Even if cancer kills me, when they autopsy my transmission they'll find it STUCK IN DRIVE.

Creating your own future is exciting. It colors each day and brings laser focus to unseen things that matter, not the seen things that do not. I am well aware my future is not about me or to be used for selfish ambition. I am always asked how many books have sold and how much money I've made. My answer is always, "I have given away more than I'll ever sell."

By this testing of my faith, I started with a snowball the size of a mustard seed and the "forward-ho" approach of Charles. We were snowballed and run over by the most powerful force in the Universe. I pray it now runs you over, too.

Warrior Words – Dorothy

Guess what cancer does? It turns you and your family inside out. Yet you cannot allow it to take over. In the 1950s it was a dirty word – you have what? The thought was pain and death with very few survivors.

Today, we have research, drugs and very caring doctors to help patients live fruitful lives. Cancer does not make you different from others. You are the same body and soul. The disease eats away at the body of both the holder of the disease and the caregiver. Stress heaps more on the brain than you realize, so at the end of the day both of us are tired, *but we do not give up!*

Life changes, with surgery, chemo, radiations and doctor appointments. Charles has plowed through five different cancers and is still up and on the road. It is slow and tough, but he has faith that it will be all right. He has never lost his sense of humor or wonderful laugh.

In caring for him I have never believed he would not get better. My degree is in nursing and we have been lucky to be able to treat bad days and rejoice in the good ones. We love each other and trust God will watch over us.

-Dorothy

CHAPTER 13
To See Another Goal

What cancer underestimates:

The depth of our faith and our hope, and the strength of a warrior's heart.

The power of goals set in a forward-thinking mind.

The strength of a human's will to live, powered by God's unwavering Holy Spirit.

The good that will be realized in spite of its evil curse.

The power of future hope and the encouragement received from another sunrise.

The compassion, strength and the unconditional love bond of a mighty caregiver.

The pure light, shining into its darkness, which gives strength and hope to heal.

The power in the written word of truth.

Cancer whispers to the warrior, "You're not strong enough to withstand the storm." The warrior shouts in reply: *"I AM THE STORM!"*

As this latest book's ride comes to an end, I am humbled again to realize what God has done for me and my family. I give Him all the credit for everything.

I pray I have offered you something – maybe just one thing. (If nothing else, I have taught you some new "F-words," or "F-bombs," as my friend would say). I trust you will find something that will be of benefit and equip you for a fuller life, now that you're out of your own way.

My hope, from one warrior to another warrior, is this: That you become more aware and have a clearer view into the darkness of this world. Whether you believe it or not, an unseen war is real, and the darkness wants to steal, kill and destroy you and your family. As Dio would say, "LOOK OUT!"

Cancer warriors, I urge you to engage with what you have been given. You may think, *I can't help.* You're wrong! Cancer people need cancer people. Never miss the opportunity to befriend another warrior. It brings healing to both and proves the good that only cancer can bring.

It is up to you to decide whether to engage in the fight, or stay home and blow your pity party horn to yourself. You must be "in it to win it" or you won't last long. If you don't engage, then stay the hell out of our way, because we "undefeated" cancer warriors, whether in treatment, out of treatment or anywhere in-between, have a new life to share and enjoy.

I urge you to continue to do your part to fund research. That's part of the fight. Last year, Sandi and I were involved in a number of American Cancer Society Relay for Life events, a Susan G. Komen conference and walk, and the National Hope Summit by the LUN-Gevity Foundation. I have spoken at the the Genentech (Tarceva® maker) annual West Coast conference. And I've donated a percent-age of each book purchase to research, and listed the names of the foundations we support at www.authorjimmorison.com.

TO SEE ANOTHER GOAL!

Don't even think for one minute goals are old hat to me. No way! I have a future list (no bucket list for me) listing my goals and dreams, and God willing I will accomplish them all. As I complete the writing of this book, I am overflowing with anticipation as I look forward to my newest, very exciting goal. Jeff and Steph will soon reveal our new grandchild. Boy am I excited – and I'm sure it's a boy.

Jenna, who you met at the beginning, is now 20 months and melts me. Every time she says "Papa" I am reminded again how very fortunate I am to share time with her. My hope for a baby boy is founded on the fact that we need to carry on the Morrison name. And Jeff needs a son

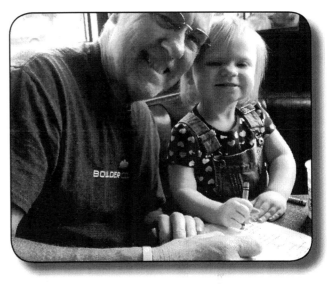

to take hunting. Onward to the maternity room I will go to meet the next impossible, beautiful goal. Once again, I am overwhelmed by grace, knowing what God has done for this ordinary blue-collar guy.

It was 11 years ago in July when I held my first grandson, soon after the surgery to remove my left lung. It was a feat that, according to man's percentages, I could never have accomplished. I thank God for making the impossible wonderful. That feeling of holding Byron against my chest was a true miracle.

So what big plans are next on my future list?

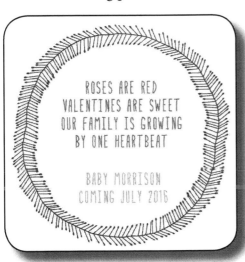

ROSES ARE RED
VALENTINES ARE SWEET
OUR FAMILY IS GROWING
BY ONE HEARTBEAT

BABY MORRISON
COMING JULY 2016

I am counting down to this coming July, when I will hug and kiss new life, which the Author of All has created and bestowed upon us. This birth will take place in new surroundings. Since Jenna was born, our Kootenai Health facility completed a beautiful addition including a new maternity department.

I will miss the second floor maternity/ICU in the old section, where I fought all those battles gone by. But all that's in my past now, and it's only fitting for my new grandchild and myself to experience new life in a new facility.

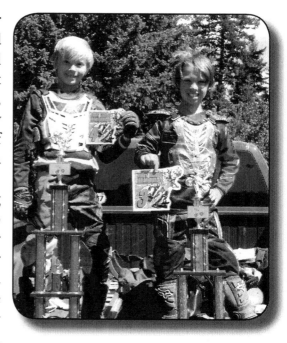

My bird-hunting gang will be heading back to Alberta in September to witness yet another sunrise from a bird blind in a pea field. I have a mule deer hunt planned for November. Our family will be fishing the derbies, towing tubes and swimming hard all summer. Byron and Carter will ride challenging trails on motorcycles.

Sandi and I will continue to travel, and try our best to keep up with a very busy family. We will enjoy the fresh garden products Chuck supplies. We will continue to try to lose weight and be healthy,

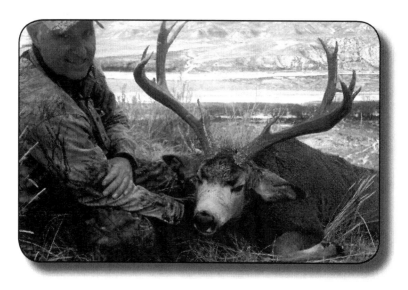

so I can keep up with Charles on our walks. It's all good and we are blessed indeed.

I will also be busy with speaking engagements and book signing trips, going to British Columbia, Washington, D.C. and San Francisco. I will be working with national, state and community cancer groups to reach out and encourage others. And always and most important, I am looking forward to the next warrior who will touch my life and remind me to thank God again for sparing my life.

I will continue to write long notes (I don't trust my chemo brain) and take pictures. You never know, I might share this next round of life with you someday soon. I hope you've been inspired, as I have, by these fellow warriors who show us what faith, goals, hope and teamwork can accomplish.

WHAT IF?

What if every person alive was a cancer survivor or a survivor of cancer? What if they had weathered cancer of their own or that of a close loved one?

Most of us, perhaps not all, would use their blessing to impact this world with common sense and hope not seen for a long time. We might again hold sacred things, well, sacred. We might honor and teach our children traditional values including God, family, the real meaning of marriage and good hard work ethics. Then we would not be screwing around wasting time with left and right, but instead, teaching right or wrong!

If only cancer warriors lived here, our planet would be a wonderful place again. Our culture would certainly look and sound different without all the useless distractions. Every day would start with a prayer of thank you and the anticipation of a new sunrise. Hope, faith and love would carry us with a grateful heart to serve others until it was time to chase the sunset. We would be content with things that really matter and the breath God has allowed. At day's end, we would rest in peace, knowing all things are possible and God has a plan.

TOO SMALL A PRICE

What good is a book if you learn nothing and feel nothing? A good book should force you to think deeply. A strong book should cut to the marrow and penetrate your joints like a double-edged sword. You should feel it judge the motives and intentions of your heart. Maybe a good book even makes you squirm a little while you're reading it. A good book reads you.

I opened such a book, in my most desperate hour, and found the story of Daniel and his three warrior buddies. Their story was pressed into my soul by the Author of Life. He prepared my heart and renewed my mind to move forward by faith, not sight, through the valley of death. My Bible challenged me not to depend on myself, or anything this world offers, and taught me that I am powerless on my own.

I have followed His light to the hill I have chosen, and I climb that hill on hands and knees. I find that the closer I get to His cross, the smaller the crowd becomes. Now in awesome wonder, speechless and pride-less, I hug the foot of that cross. I look up and meet the radiant light that He showed us in the blazing furnace. *I was blind but now I see. I have paid too small a price for all my sins, since he did nothing wrong.*

As overwhelmed as I am by His light at the cross, how much more will I be by His power over the empty grave? From tragedy to triumph, he rescued me, just as He promised. *(Daniel 3:16-18) And now I know that triumph can only come with tragedy. Darkness lost again! And will forever!*

I know in whom I have believed. By His resurrection power that resides in me, I was made able to break the chains of captivity that cancer held tight. From my evil pit of despair, I journeyed into the light of the most beautiful rainbow my Lord has ever created. *My life matters to him! So does yours!*

Now freed from cancer's darkness and sin's stranglehold, my conduct must reflect my new allegiance. And so must my writing.

I invite you, my fellow warriors and all others in need of rescue, to accept God's plan for your life. Only when you move forward in

His will, not your own, does life once again have value and the course of action becomes clear. There is no other way.

I have included a page for Your Response at the end of this book. I urge you to pick your hill and be resolved. *(Daniel 1:8)* Please, don't delay. Fill it out and then e-mail me so we can rejoice together.

Thank God my own major storm has long passed. I remain even stronger now with His mighty power in me. I can stand firm, armored with God's truth, rooted deep in the things this wicked culture cannot see and refuses to understand.

Today, I devote my extended time to chasing goals, sunsets, grandchildren and mule deer, while all the time knowing that my real job is holding a shield of comfort over fellow warriors and caregivers when their own storm rolls its darkness overhead and calls their name. I share the light, so they too may stand their ground.

Thank you for reading this book. Thank you for allowing me to share my life's battles and those of my fellow warriors. I am honored to have your attention and support. I pray you have goals that are every bit as exciting to you as mine are to me.

May the God of Light and Creation touch and bless you.

Let the Son-rise shine! It is finished!

Advice For Caregivers

YOUR ROLE AS CAREGIVER FOR A CANCER PATIENT

As your loved one's caregiver, you may fill many roles and have many responsibilities. You are important. You are needed. And your attention and involvement can make a big difference in your loved one's care; too many patients lack someone like you in their lives.

WHAT DOES IT MEAN TO BE AN "ACTIVE PARTICIPANT" IN YOUR LOVED ONE'S CARE?

It's important that a caregiver be a part of the team from the very beginning. That means you can help your loved one make decisions, plan treatment, and follow treatment instructions carefully.

To do this, you will need to be as informed as possible. Having the care team's perspective as well as your loved one's point of view can allow you to truly be the advocate you need to be.

WHAT RESPONSIBILITIES CAN YOU EXPECT?

Trying to learn how to help someone with cancer? As a caregiver, you may have many responsibilities for managing your loved one's overall care, including:
- monitoring and writing down health needs
- encouraging emotional well-being
- helping your loved one follow treatments and make healthy lifestyle changes
- managing insurance claims and bill payments

Serving as an advocate means you give voice to your loved one's needs and wishes. This may include:

- informing the care team of any changes, new symptoms or side effects, and asking for help in managing them
- locating hard-to-find information
- encouraging your loved one to speak up about his or her wants and needs

There are different ways to help the ones you love.

BRIDGE COMMUNICATIONS

Friends, family, and community play an important role in everyone's well-being. You can help channel those communications by answering calls, sending emails, or updating a daily blog so everyone who cares is informed. You can also find ways to build meaningful connections between your loved one and family, friends, neighbors, and others.

For example, you might arrange for a favorite relative to visit for the weekend.

OFFER FRIENDSHIP OR LOVING SUPPORT

Before lung cancer, you already offered companionship to your loved one, whether as a friend or family member. Now, you might need to be around more often or make yourself more available, because your loved one really needs your support. This may mean you go from simply enjoying Sunday breakfasts together to attending medical appointments, running errands, and doing household chores.

DISCUSS TREATMENT OPTIONS WITH THE CARE TEAM AND YOUR LOVED ONE

It's important that you and your loved one discuss what is most important. Talk about what your loved one needs, establish priorities, and make sure any wishes are fully understood. Knowing these details can help ensure all discussions with the care team reflect your loved one's point of view.

Together, you might review treatment options with the care team and ask questions to ensure both you and your loved one fully understand.

CAREGIVERS NEED CARE, TOO

Learning a loved one has cancer can be devastating. Add to that the long list of duties a caregiver takes on, and the role can quickly become overwhelming. While a survey of 100 caregivers of people with cancer found that 92% reported that they found the caregiving experience to be overwhelming, the same amount found the experience to be rewarding.

"Taking the time to take care of yourself can help you be a better caregiver for your loved one," says Win Boerckel, Director of Social Service, Long Island Office at CancerCare. "It's important to know your limits and to remember that you aren't alone. Take advantage of resources and support available to you, and – most importantly – ask for and accept help."

FIND A SUPPORT TEAM

As a caregiver, you may feel alone or that no one understands. That couldn't be further from the truth.

Asking for help from YOUR support team is okay, too. You can't do it all, nor should you try. And it's fine to admit that. You'll only end up exhausted. And that won't serve you or your loved one well.

Who can you recruit for your support team? A spouse or partner, close friends and family members, neighbors, members of your faith community, even colleagues can offer timely support. Many people have been in a similar position and may welcome the chance to "pay it forward." There are also organizations that offer help to caregivers like you with services that range from counseling to free massages.

Don't wait until you're exhausted to reach out for help— start your search now.

FIND SOMEONE TO LISTEN TO YOU

As a caregiver, you might feel like you have to stay positive and strong for your loved one, but it's important to find ways to express your own feelings too. In the same survey, 55% of caregivers say that speaking with another person, such as a friend, is how they cope and 40% find connecting with other caregivers to be helpful. Online tools can help you find support groups and community services in your area.

MAINTAIN YOUR OWN HEALTH

While you may frequently find yourself in a doctor's office with your loved one, remember to keep up with your own health, too. Make appointments with your doctor/therapist as needed, and slow down if you are feeling ill. As a caregiver, your health, happiness and quality of life matter too!

ASK FOR AND ACCEPT HELP

People want to pay it forward. You can't do it all, nor should you try. Build your own support team (your spouse or partner, friends, neighbors, etc.), and ask for help before you get overwhelmed or exhausted. You can also visit online resources to find support services in your area.

TAKE A BREAK

To be a better caregiver, it's important to take a break. Different activities that get you out of the house and the clinic can work for different people. For instance, go for a walk, go out to lunch, take an exercise class at your local gym, express yourself through artwork or journaling — either in a notebook or online.

Your Response

"God, I recognize that I have not lived my life for You up until now. I have been living for myself and that is wrong. I need You in my life; I want You in my life. I acknowledge the completed work of Your Son Jesus Christ in giving His life for me on the cross at Calvary, and I long to receive the forgiveness you have made freely available to me through this sacrifice. Come into my life now, Lord. Take up residence in my heart and be my king, my Lord, and my Savior. From this day forward, I will no longer be controlled by sin, or the desire to please myself, but I will follow You all the days of my life. Those days are in Your hands. I ask this in Jesus' precious and holy name. Amen."

_____

Sign and date

Please feel free to contact me at either my email address (toseeanothersunrise@gmail.com) or via our website (www.authorjimmorrison.com) so that we may rejoice together, pray together, or share your stories.